HEALTH CARE
MANAGEMENT
IN MIND

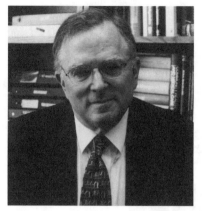**Anthony R. Kovner, PhD,** is Professor of Health Policy and Management at the Robert F. Wagner Graduate School of Public Service at New York University, in New York City. He received bachelor's and master's degrees from Cornell University, and his doctorate in public administration from the University of Pittsburgh. He is an experienced health care manager, having served as chief executive officer of a community hospital, senior health care consultant for United Autoworkers Union in Detroit, manager of a group practice, of a nursing home and of a large ambulatory care services program. He is a board member of the Lutheran Medical Center of Brooklyn, NY and Vice Chairman of the board of Health Plus. Kovner was the fourth recipient of the Gary L. Filerman prize for Educational Leadership, awarded in June 1999, by the Association of University Programs in Health Administration.

Kovner has consulted extensively in the health care industry in the areas of board development, management development, implementation of community benefit programs, and strategic planning. Some recent clients include: Montefiore Medical Center, the Oxford Health Plans, and the Clara Maass Health System.

Kovner has completed research projects on how hospitals can be governed more effectively, and how to implement management development programs for health care organizations. He is currently studying the impact of Medicaid managed care on large New York City health plans. He has carried out several demonstration programs funded by the Robert Wood Foundation and the W. K. Kellogg Foundation, and program initiatives for the Pew Charitable Trusts and the Milbank Memorial Fund.

He has written a number of books, including *Really Managing* (Health Administration Press, 1988), *A Career Guide for the Health Services Manager* (coauthored with Alan Channing; Health Administration Press, 1999), *Health Care Delivery in the United States* (Springer Publishing Co., 1999), *The Role of the Physician Executive* (coauthored with David Kindig, Health Administration Press, 1992), *Health Services Management* (coedited with Duncan Neuhauser, Health Administration Press, 1997) and *Health Services Management: A Book of Cases* (coedited with Duncan Neuhauser, Health Administration Press, 1997).

He has published articles in many journals including *Frontiers of Health Services Management, Journal of Rural Health, Journal of Health Administration Education, Hospital and Health Services Administration, Health Affairs, Inquiry, Trustee, Medical Care,* and *Health Care Management Review.*

HEALTH CARE
MANAGEMENT IN MIND

EIGHT CAREERS

ANTHONY R. KOVNER, PhD

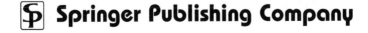 Springer Publishing Company

Copyright © 2000 by Springer Publishing Company, Inc.

Springer Publishing Company, Inc.
536 Broadway
New York, NY 10012-3955

Acquisitions Editor: Bill Tucker
Production Editor: Pamela Lankas
Cover design by James Scotto-Lavino

00 01 02 03 04 / 5 4 3 2 1

Library of Congress Cataloging-in-Publication-Data

Kovner, Anthony R.
    Health care management in mind : eight careers / Anthony R. Kovner.
        p.   cm.
    Includes bibliographical references and index.
    ISBN 0-8261-1315-X
        1. Health services administration—Vocational guidance.   I. Title.
    RA971.K647 2000
    362.1'068—dc21

                                            99-057678

Printed in the United States of America

It has been my experience, that the one quality, aside from built-in gifts, which separates the extraordinary executives from the ordinary is the pleasure they take in their work.

—Warren Bennis

For My Grandchildren

Contents

Preface   *ix*

Foreword by James Knickman   *xi*

1   What My Grandfathers Did   1

2   Managing the Family Business   11

3   Managing Health Care for the Poor   23

4   Managing in Academia   39

5   Laboring for the Union   55

6   Hospital Chief Executive, But Not for Long   67

7   Consultant to Large Foundations   79

8   Governing Nonprofits   97

9   Managing in Academia: A Reprise   115

10 Lessons Learned in Eight Careers   137

Afterword by Duncan Neuhauser   *145*

References   *149*

Index   *153*

Note: Some of the names used in the text are fictionalized—for example, Will Jonas and Dr. Flux in chapter 3, all the protagonists and the name of the town in chapter 6, and the names of the three organizations to which I consulted, in chapter 8. In the cases of the individuals, this was done to preserve privacy, and in the case of the organizations, because mine was only a partial view of what was actually going on.

Preface

This book is meant for those who teach, do research, and practice health care, and for those who govern and manage nonprofit organizations. I started writing this when, at the age of 61, I realized that I had not told my children, 26 and 24, about my life at work, and when I realized that I was ignorant about what my grandfathers did. I didn't feel I wanted to share with anyone the truth about my life, but I wanted to write a personal and truthful, insofar as I could make it, account of my life at work. This book is the result.

I sent the manuscript to two friends, Duncan Neuhauser, professor of Health Management at Case Western Reserve University, and Rob Fromberg, associate director of the Health Administration Press. Both encouraged me to seek publication. Bill Tucker and Ursula Springer at Springer Publishing accepted the manuscript, and suggested that I add short sections to each chapter, making specific suggestions to help managers apply what I had learned to their own situations.

I have tried to tell it like it was. I hope some of the lessons that I have learned can help managers make more of themselves than would otherwise be the case. Of course, observations from the field always have the potential to contradict what one has read or been told. But such events emphasize the resourcefulness of the individual and the range of capability of the manager (Lopez, 1986).

A colleague at NYU's Wagner School, Dennis Smith, suggested that I add a word about my values. In my June 1999 acceptance speech for the Gary L. Filerman Prize for Educational Leadership from the Association of University Programs in Health Administration, I shared with the audience my values as a teacher and practitioner of health care management: (a) national health insurance for all Americans, (b) market capitalism, (c) health care organizations as community organizations, and (d) putting the customer first, in health care and in education for health care management. More about this, both rationale and explanation, in the pages that follow.

In addition to those already named in this Preface, I would like to acknowledge the contributions of commentators on the original manuscript: Steven Finkler, Jack Karp, James Knickman, Victor Kovner, Anna Kovner, Ruth Krall, Michael Rosenthal, and Dennis Smith.

Special thanks to Sarah Christine Kovner, for her superb editing of the entire manuscript.

Reference

Lopez, B. (1986). *Arctic dreams.* New York: Scribner's.

Foreword

Health Care Management in Mind is a book unlike any you have read. I have read it three times at this point. Each time, I finished the book in one sitting because I could not get myself to put it down. And, each time I feel like I have read a different book. This, it turns out, is by design because Tony Kovner has managed to weave together three incredibly engaging topics in this one, short book.

The first reading of the book—and the most important one to me—is as a biography. Kovner has had a fascinating, varied career in health care management and academe. He has made many important contributions as a leader and a researcher, but his career—like those of most of us—has not always been 100% successful or glamorous. This biography—which is mostly professional rather than personal—is starkly frank and self-critical, and always informative and educational.

What can you say about somebody who is willing to describe being fired in one way or another four times in his life? What do you say about somebody willing to tell his story for two key reasons: First, to leave behind a record for his children and hoped-for grandchildren who he thinks can learn from his experience and second, to provide educational materials for students of management? A very special person emerges from these pages; a person who learns slowly but surely from his experiences, a person dedicated to the field of health care and the field of management, a person with firm values and perseverance.

The second reading of this book, which I hardly noticed during the first read, focused on the management lessons that emerged from each professional position Tony held. By the end of career number 8, a comprehensive set of management issues and lessons are evident in this biography. At the end of each chapter, Kovner provides a context for how students can learn from his experiences. And, each chapter works as an excellent case study considering issues in health care management and the delivery and organization of health care.

The third reading of the book highlighted a selective history of the health policy and management field. As part of each section, Kovner provides useful commentary on the issues of the day that were relevant to the management job he held at the time. Some of these issues are about public policy and some are about broader social or delivery issues facing the health sector. As such, the book works as a very readable history of some important challenges the health care industry has faced over the past 30 years.

Because this is a personal book, I think it fair to relate two anecdotes about working with Tony. I have worked with Tony in one way or another for almost 20 years and suggest the following stories to help readers understand the author and the book.

One of the first times I worked with Tony was on a curriculum committee to redesign a statistics course at NYU (a topic Tony should have known very little about). He had just joined the NYU faculty, and at this first meeting he quickly announced that I should be the chair of the curriculum committee and that he would be the secretary and keep the notes. After about 5 minutes of discussion, he announced that he had finished the notes and was pleased that we had come to agreement so quickly! I had my first lesson in management from Professor Kovner: Take the initiative and be sure to take the notes! Readers will see that Kovner has taken notes that are useful for all of us throughout his professional career.

My second personal story also dates back to early encounters with Kovner as an NYU faculty member. An avid squash player with no partners, the new faculty member insisted that we play squash together. After a few minutes of practice that made it clear he was in a different league in terms of skills, Tony announced we should start the game; a score of 21 would win, and I could start with a handicap of 19 points. This was management lesson number 2: Count on your opponent to play at full speed and set the rules so you always are pushed to perform at your best.

Many mutual acquaintances insist that Tony and I should have hated each other from start to end. We come from different backgrounds, do very different types of research, and have very different styles of day-to-day coping with what life brings us. However, this book makes clear why Tony is such a valued friend and colleague. His honesty, his striving to make a difference in a complex world, his willingness to learn from the past, and his willingness to open himself up to help others learn from what he does: these are rare traits in a person and in a friend. Readers of this book will benefit from his experience.

JAMES R. KNICKMAN

1

What My Grandfathers Did

In this first chapter I provide an overview to the succeeding chapters, discuss some lessons learned about health care management and nonprofit governance, and introduce my family history, as this is relevant to my eight careers.

Lessons Learned about Health Care Management

Health care management is similar in some respects to management of services in education, social services, art, and religion. Outputs are not easily measurable and service providers are highly professionalized. Since 1990, the health care industry has changed in two important ways. The industry is rapidly becoming more concentrated as larger firms become vertically integrated. Second, more of the industry is for-profit, and more large, for-profit firms have merged to become huge organizations, for example, Aetna and US Health Care, Cigna, Beverly Enterprises, or HealthSouth. This concentration has the following effects: the managerial role becomes more critical for organizational effectiveness, more physicians choose to become managers, and health care managers become more like managers in the for-profit sector.

Is this good for the patient? Or as my father used to say "Is this good for the Jews?" Similar variance occurs among for-profit firms and not-for-profit firms. The same for-profit physicians who provided too many services under fee-for-service reimbursement supply too few under capitation payment, while larger organizations allow for economies of scale and specialization of function, such as quality improvement, which may or may not improve outcomes for patients.

Thousands of management jobs exist in health care. Yet, many practicing managers lack the skills and experience now in demand. For example, today's health care managers must be familiar with the performance indicators necessary to evaluate health care delivery and with the best practices in quality improvement, operations management, governance information systems, cost accounting, marketing, team building and management development. The discrepancy between needed skills and experienced managers is due to differences in training, a failure to keep abreast of the state of the field, and the failure of organizations to invest in the future of their managers.

I tell my masters' students that if they are willing to work hard and are able to get along well with others, they will be ahead of 50% of their competition. Most important are the outcomes to which managers contribute and take responsibility for. These outcomes include increasing revenue, improving quality, improving access, or decreasing unit costs. Managers must be seen as trustworthy by their bosses, subordinates, and peers. Networking is important, and helping others so that they will help you. Reflecting on your own management practice can assist in continually thinking about how the manager spends and should spend scarce time and presence in focusing upon results.

No organizational or managerial accountability can exist without specification of measurable objectives. These objectives then should be shared and validated by those with a stake in organizational performance. Managers learn by listening, and they must give the appearance of listening. To be perceived as adding value, managers should be experts in some area or domain. The natural areas for nonclinical expertise are finance, information, operations and marketing. Communication skills are paramount—being able to read and write, listen and speak effectively. Another important skill is the ability to know when there is something you don't know and where to or how to better define the question.

To bring about change, managers must first be able to "ruthlessly" describe a current situation, then analyze the problems and issues which flow from that situation. They must also be able to come up with inexpensive solutions that are aligned with the interests of those in power, for change does not come about unless those in power become convinced that change is in their interest.

Lessons Learned About Nonprofit Governance

Nonprofit is similar to for-profit governance (Pointer & Orlikoff, 1999)[1] (where there is also a board of directors), and to governmental governance

---

[1] According to Pointer and Orlikoff, the essence of governing is: formulating policy, making decisions, engaging in oversight with respect to ends, executive management performance, quality of care, finances, and their own practices.

(where the legislative branch performs oversight of the executive). The difference lies in the construction of the accountability structure. For-profit directors are elected by shareholders. The criteria for organizational performance is profit, market share, return on invested capital, now or over a longer term. In government, legislators are elected by the voters and there is no agreed upon criterion of performance (other than being responsive to the preferences of voters and interest groups who provide candidates with funding and information so that they can seek election and reelection). The main challenge for nonprofit governance is account-ability, as boards of directors are usually elected by themselves, often with no term or age limits.

Nonprofits' lack of accountability is counterbalanced by the importance of mission. Mission is the reason donors give, employees work, and participants use the services of nonprofits, be it a church, a museum, or a health care organization. The board should be the conscience of an organization, building in safeguards to see that the original mission is adhered to, or that it is consciously and deliberately altered consonant with the spirit of the original mission but in response to changed circumstances. External pressures and constraints, such as government regulation and the articulated preferences of demanding consumers, can serve to keep the board's feet to the fire. All these elements are often lacking in nonprofits, not to mention that there is often conflict of interest among, or benign neglect by, board members.

In my experience, the main challenge in nonprofit governance is convincing those who dominate the board that it is in their interest to improve organizational and board performance to carry out the imperatives of mission. After all, it is the nonprofit form, perhaps more than anything else, which has sustained democratic pluralism in our great country. Nonprofits have achieved tremendous results in education, health care, social welfare, and the arts, sectors not supported to the same extent in other countries. It is difficult for board members to change behavior and revitalize mission for several reasons: (1) they think they are doing good which ought to convince others that they are doing their job. Some board members give and contribute money and time, and besides, they aren't being paid for board service; (2) board members are most comfortable working with people like themselves—usually people who are wealthy, white, male, age 55+, usually businessmen, bankers, and lawyers by profession; (3) since the board is responsible for the way things are in a nonprofit, board members are, almost by definition comfortable with the status quo, and making changes takes time and effort. Significant change, moreover, involves political risk and often personal discomfort in facing difficult people and difficult issues, which is not why most people join boards. And besides, the organization is currently carrying out its mission, money is being raised, people are being served, and if the organization is not doing better, this is often for reasons beyond the board's or management's control, such as government cutbacks or union demands.

There is nothing magical about what makes for an effective board; this requires leadership and vision. From experience, I have become convinced that leadership and vision are much more important than the function, structure, and composition of the board—the subject of most academic research. The most effective form of leadership consists of a respected leader, usually the board chair, primarily advised and supported by an inner ring of trusted, somewhat diverse, advisor board members, who have excellent communication with a still more diverse outer ring of board members and organizational stakeholders. Effective boards can come in many forms: large, nondiverse, paid, and with or absent chief executives as board members. Board meetings can be held monthly, quarterly, or annually; effective boards can have annual, or less frequent, retreats or not. I have my views on all these matters, but again the key question is how on a board of trustees to generate and retain effective leadership and vision.

There isn't any specific recipe for leadership and vision. Nor should nonprofit organizations have any permanence or longevity substantially different from that of for-profits. Organizations are temporary relative to societies and are justified based on the value they add to the inputs supplied by the greater society. When a nonprofit ceases to add value relative to alternative uses of the inputs, it no longer deserves to exist. What I mean to suggest here is that those considering joining a board or changing a board must carefully interpret the given situation. I have always divided up issues and problems requiring intervention as falling into three piles: (a) important but the intervenor cannot do anything about it; (b) unimportant and not worth the intervenor's time and energy; and (c) important and worth getting involved with. So I recommend only joining a board with the requisite leadership and vision. As a member of a board lacking the same, I would discuss with the leadership what I think needs to be done. If I saw no signs of appropriate progress I would resign and explain my reasons for doing so.

My action would be no different as a scholar concerned with studying such governance, a consultant aiming to improve board performance, or a board member of a poorly performing board who has a loyalty or commitment to the organization because of historic or personal relationships, or for other reasons. Scholars should pay more attention to the factors promoting leadership and vision—how can these factors be measured, and what are the differences in processes as well as outcomes in organizations with and without boards with requisite leadership and vision? Consultants, who are usually primarily concerned with generating their own revenues, should see the surest way to attract future business is working with boards where the consultant can add considerable value and show results. As far as remaining on a poorly performing board, this should be a conscious choice as a consumption rather than an investment activity; in other words, the involved board member should acknowledge that little or nothing can be done to improve performance but accept that he or she wishes to remain and continue on the board for other reasons.

What do I mean by boards having the requisite leadership and vision? The leader must be able to transform (Burns, 1978) followers so that their energy is liberated and focused in pursuit of the mission. The leader is able to do this because he or she is trusted, can generate resources, or because followers believe that the leader takes their preferences into consideration. The leader understands the business of the nonprofit and can objectively determine, with the help of others, the characteristics of an excellent delivery system, whether this is art, education, health care, or religion. He or she can compare excellence with present circumstances, articulate the problems and issues which present circumstances raise, and identify realistic and aligned recommendations to improve board and organizational performance. Many would argue, which I do not deny, that this is the responsibility of the chief executive. Yet, where the board adds value is in its focus on longer term issues, whereas an executive must be fully immersed in the present. The board should be the conscience of the organization, buffered from the personal interests of the chief executive, whether this is in terms of power, money, or policy.

This brings us to the concepts of "vision" and "mission." For me, the difference between the two words is that *mission* implies values while *vision* implies strategy. This is not to follow Alice in Wonderland where the Queen says that words mean what she says they do. A nonprofit mission must be seen as having value in the greater society, at least by those who provide the organization with resources and legitimacy. Vision, however, involves figuring out the niche of the nonprofit where it can add the most value relative to competing organizations, whether this concerns who is served, what the service is, or how the service is delivered. Any board mission and vision needs to be articulated and validated with external and internal stakeholders, a long and costly process. From my own experience, most boards are not up to doing this properly. Reasonable stakeholders will not necessarily agree about mission and vision, particularly as this involves resource trade-offs. But a certain amount of change is to be desired by any effective nonprofit: (1) this includes change in the powers that be, (2) changes in policy preferences, and (3) even changes in mission and vision since the society and its organizational stakeholders also change over time.

My Eight Careers

Most of this book is about health care management and nonprofit governance. It's based on my eight careers. Nine chapters follow this one, the last chapter summing up some views on managing your career, life and work, and the effective manager. In over 40 years, I have worked with a rich variety of health care and other organizations. For the purpose of this volume, my eight careers are: (1) for-profit manager in a family-owned health care business, (2) manager of a large urban neighborhood health center, (3 & 4) management professor and health care administration program director (twice), (5) union senior health care consultant, (6) consultant to large private foundations, (7) hospital manager, and (8) nonprofit board member. The time period of my eight careers starts with my graduation from Cornell University in 1957 and ends in 1997, some 40 years later. (As of July 1999, I am still employed as a professor at New York University.)

Any of the careers just described could have been full time (although a career as a nonprofit board member would require other paid employment). At least half of my career has been spent as a professor, during which time I have also held various managerial positions, that is, I was director of our school's health program for 10 years. During 40 years, I have spent a great deal of time consulting, writing, and serving on boards. I have lived, worked, and consulted in most of the states in the continental United States and in a few countries overseas. My full-time positions have been in the greater New York City area, the greater Philadelphia/ Southern New Jersey area, and in Detroit. Additionally, I was a student for several years in Ithaca, NY, and in Pittsburgh, PA.

Some of the central issues in which I am most interested are national health insurance, accountability of nonprofits, management of nonprofits, and research on the management and governance of health care organizations. Health insurance coverage is the most important health care issue affecting Americans today, even though the 40 million Americans without health insurance get 60% of the services that Americans with health insurance get, which represents more expenditures per capita than those in any other country in the world. The issue is still critical. Then, the question becomes how best to insure all Americans; or put another way, what form of national health insurance for all Americans has the least dysfunctional consequences? Such consequences include: too much government power, lack of innovation, waste of money, and diluting the quality of our physicians, hospitals, and our research on medical and health services delivery.

The lack of accountability of nonprofits is another serious issue. More nonprofits with more resources do more good in America than in any other country in the world. They serve as a check on government power and as a vehicle for the rich to support charitable purposes. Would the government really spend the money better and achieve more results than do the nonprofit organizations? Would the country be better off with only government and for-profit organizations, operating in the education, health care, social welfare, and religious sectors? The question, I think, is how best to facilitate and encourage appropriate accountability from the nonprofit sector? For example, nonprofit boards can be subject to the same constraints, with regard to public disclosure, as for-profits. There is more agreement on the desirability of greater accountability for nonprofits than there is agreement about how such accountability should be specified, and what, if any, sanctions, should be enforced if greater accountability is lacking. Surely, governmental intrusion should be minimized. Previously, I have suggested boards sharing organizational objectives with and reporting on progress to external and internal stakeholders. Implementing these solutions requires significant investments both in time and money to carry out effectively. Boards, for the most part, have not seen it as in their interest to arrange for and monitor such processes.

Because significant change is *not* usually *in* the interest of many of the powers that control nonprofits, it is not strange that they do not see significant change as desirable. The powers that be in any organization have made a significant investment which they do not want to risk losing. It is most efficient for them to keep things the way they are, particularly when the side payments to board members for getting involved in change are usually slight. Part of the problem relates to the costs and benefits of getting rid of the powers that be, relative to starting all over. The easiest way to get significant change accomplished quickly in any nonprofit is to hire new people whose own ideas and commitments are to make the changes. And what does this signify (where is the justice?) for those who have worked hard to do the best that they can under different rules and different circumstances? But where is the justice in these people not acquiring the new skills, experience, and values required for different times and circumstances?

Other than the researchers, few care about management and governance research. It's not that this research can't be done or shouldn't be done, it's that no one wants to pay as yet significant dollars to see such research accomplished. Commitment to carrying out management and governance research, especially in health care and nonprofit organizations, requires a longer time perspective than most service organizations have, and diverts funds away from service. To get this kind of research funded, somebody has to do it on the cheap, or on a pilot basis, or, what is more difficult, prove to or persuade others that the benefits of the research outweigh the costs and have a priority relative to other uses of the funds.

My Family History

In managing your own career, I have found it useful to speculate about how your parents came to be what they turned out to be. First, this frames any advice they may wish to give you. Second, it forces you to examine what they did and to ask yourself how you can learn from their experience. All that I know about my grandparents is that on my father's side, Louis Kovner escaped from Russia to avoid having to serve in the Russian army. Louis, apparently a dashing young man, was rescued by women and emigrated to the United States at the turn of the century. Subsequently, he worked as a peddler, then in the paper box business. Once in New York, he moved to Brooklyn and became a real estate speculator, married, with four children. His wife Anna died young, before I was born. Louis' son, Sidney, my father, was born in Brooklyn in 1904. A star athlete in high school, he attended the Wharton undergraduate program in business at the University of Pennsylvania. Upon graduation, he went into business with his father and his brother, Harold.

On my mother's side, both her parents immigrated to the United States from middle-European countries at about the same time as my paternal grandfather. Percy Behrman attended NYU medical school in the early 1900s, and became a family physician. Due to his contraction of tuberculosis, he moved to rural southern New Jersey with his family. His wife, Eva, was a housewife and stage mother. My mother, Natalie, one of three children, received scholarships to the Juilliard School of Music and to the Theater Guild of Acting. She was a child performer on the New York stage, performed in the Yiddish theater, and won a New York City beauty contest as a teenager.

My parents were divorced in 1946, and subsequently married Europeans who were very physically attractive and younger than they. My brother and I lived with my mother. My father and his new wife had a daughter, my sister, Kiki, in 1951. My father wanted me to work with him in the family business. He never made a big point of this—it was more or less assumed. My mother wanted me to go to medical school, but if not to medical school, then to law school. My father said it was not necessary, to go into his business. And so, the story begins.

Reflection: Learning from Your Parents

My father went into business to make money and to live the high life. My mother developed a charitable foundation because she needed something to do which fit her self image as a woman who deserved to be with rich and influential persons. Consider the following situations:

1. Sarah Yin's immigrant parents fled dictatorship and poverty and operate a laundromat. They want her to marry a fellow national who is a physician. Sarah is pursuing her degree in health care management and wants to manage a nursing home.

2. Tony Ruffino's father was a postal carrier and his mother, a housewife. Tony worked as a financial officer in a bank, and has enrolled in a health care management program because he wants to work for an organization with a strong sense of mission rather than one that is primarily profit-driven. Tony's parents say that he should do whatever he wants to do.

3. Bill Greenberg's father was a physician and his mother, a lawyer. Bill likes being a physician, but he is making less money and getting less satisfaction from being an obstetrician-gynecologist than he thought he would. His father thinks Bill should stay a physician because this is what he knows and who he is.

What can you learn from these examples? The earlier the manager decides on a health care management career, the more efficient his/her career path. On the other hand, younger people have the opportunity to try different things, to learn from experience, with a resultant fuller appreciation of any final choice. The imperative is, at some time, for managers to spend enough time in focused pursuit of what it is they want to do. This requires two steps: (1) talking to people who are managers to get more accurate information about various jobs and about yourself as others see you; and, (2) developing the competencies and contacts necessary to pursue a managerial career.

My parents gave me good advice—to make money, and to work hard. However, I didn't spend enough time thinking about what they didn't tell me. My father wanted me to help him in his business, which was the wrong advice for me. My mom wanted me *not* to be like my father, to become a physician like her father, which I successfully resisted. In retrospect, I can see that I should have taken charge of my life earlier, focused on future job opportunities, and on managing my career. Despite my relative success, I would advise a different strategy for those entering the management field. You can accomplish more in less time.

Learning From Your Parents: A Checklist

Yes	No	
_____	_____	Do you understand what your parents want for you and why they want it for you?
_____	_____	Do you understand what you want for yourself at work?
_____	_____	Have you sought out persons who have the kinds of jobs you think you would like to have?
_____	_____	Have you found out from these individuals what they like about their jobs, and what it really takes to succeed at their jobs?
_____	_____	Have you tried to understand what your parents haven't told you about the career decisions that they made and why they made them?
_____	_____	In what ways are you different from your parents, and what does this imply about your career decisions?
_____	_____	Have you taken responsibility for managing your career now, and what are you doing about it?

Practical Exercise

Write a memo to yourself indicating how your parents have helped you to get where you are now, with regard to your skills, experience and values. Specify how their career goals for you differ from yours. Explain how you can deal with any of their objections to doing what it is you most want to do in your career.

2

Managing the Family Business

In 1957, my father and uncle owned five small institutions: two for-profit hospitals in New York City (The Park East and the Park West), a hospital and a nursing home in the Bronx, and a sanatorium (former TB hospital) in Morristown, NJ. Most of the doctors who admitted to the Park East, where my father and uncle shared a large office, had practices near the hospital, and many of them sent most of their admissions to the larger and more prestigious Mount Sinai Hospital about a mile away. The Park East's main competitor, Doctors' Hospital, a similar, small hospital was about one-half mile away. In 1957, there were many small hospitals in the city, and many of them did quite well.

The Park East Hospital

The Park East Hospital had 116 beds and was about nine stories high. It had been built as a hospital by a physician owner. My father, uncle, and grandfather bought the two Manhattan hospitals from this doctor during the Depression as real estate and found themselves having to run, rather than sell, them. The former owner, a physician, died shortly thereafter. The hospitals were beneficiaries under his insurance policies, and the money which was sizeable, came in handy during difficult times.

What I remember about the Park East Hospital (it is now an apartment house) was the elegant lobby of comfortable sofas and paintings (my uncle was an art collector who supported artists) and the telephone alcove on the right, complete with switchboards. One of my cousins

11

worked there one summer as a teenage switchboard operator. The patient rooms upstairs were very comfortable. I was born at the Park East, and was once a patient there at age 27 (for a tonsillectomy). Many of the nurses worked there for many years, and they were always very friendly and took care of me. And then, of course, my father, Sidney, and my uncle, Harold, three years older, occupied the large office on the second floor.

This office was like a stage set in a farce. People kept entering and leaving. My father and uncle did business together, or separately, from behind their huge desks. The room had a large television set and a sofa, large, colorful paintings, and black and white family photographs. My father arranged to be shaved and have his hair trimmed every day by his barber, Julius, who had a shop down the street. The business that the Kovner brothers conducted there, so far as I could tell, had little to do with hospitals. Regular attendees were Murray Singer, the business accountant (who when I was a child used to place the rings off his cigars around my small fingers) and Mickey Silvers, the family bookie, who was also my father's longtime handball partner, and companion for crap games and women. Also present were a troop of doctors, artists, persons seeking loans or jobs, and family and friends. Uncle Harold, an amateur psychiatrist who held a law degree, was a professional womanizer. My father was an inveterate gambler, both in the stock market and on football, baseball, and basketball games. He was in constant touch by phone with his stockbroker.

Growing Up

I was brought up as a rich man's child. We lived in an apartment on Park Avenue, and always had a governess and maid. My father had a chauffeur. I attended private school with my cousin Victor, Harold's son, who is six months younger than I. Victor never wanted to go into the family business. For some reason, which is still largely inexplicable to me, I never gave the matter of what I would do for a living any thought while I was growing up. I never discussed my future career with my parents. My father told me that I should go to college and have a good time, and after that "we would worry about it."

If I was not thinking about what I was going to do when I grew up, what was I thinking about? During high school (where I was two years younger than my classmates, having skipped a grade during elementary school and having started early) I was smaller than everyone else and less sophisticated. As I remember it now, 45 years later, I was involved during my senior year of high school in a great romance with a sophomore in high school, who subsequently left me for a college student from Ohio State. In short, high school was a time to dream about girls, to watch and play sports, and to read a lot of novels. My mother wanted me to go to Harvard, Yale, or Princeton, but I couldn't get in. Then she wanted me to sit out a year, go to prep school, and apply again, but I rejected her advice. My father wanted me to go to Penn, where he had gone to the Wharton School. But I applied to Cornell because it had been recommended to me as a good school that was not so far away, and I was accepted. Following my father's advice, I enrolled in ROTC, Reserve Officer's Training Corps in the Army, and I took courses in Accounting and Insurance, although I majored in English Literature. I thought I was majoring in Literature, but learned too late that this was *English* Literature, which meant I would be reading British poets rather than European and American novelists.

After graduating from Cornell, I served in the army. During the summer of my junior year, my ROTC class had been stationed in Fort Bragg, North Carolina, where I was persistently behind everyone in military skills, especially in being able to take apart, reassemble, and keep my M-1 rifle neat and shiny. As part of the training, we had to fire machine guns, after which my ear started and never stopped ringing. I went to the doctor, and was told that if I didn't sign a paper saying I was okay, I wouldn't be allowed to leave Fort Bragg. So I signed and left. My hearing was permanently damaged; I can't hear my watch ticking in my left ear, but I don't wear a hearing aid. I never sued anyone and, of course, I was subsequently assigned to the air defense artillery, in El Paso, Texas.

At Fort Bliss, we had to wear uniforms and attend classes every day from 9 AM to 5 PM. This was a big switch from college, where we attended classes (only if we chose) 15 hours a week. When the officers fired the antiaircraft 90 millimeter guns, I stayed home, with a doctor's note. For each hourly class, we were given a lesson plan which the military instructor followed, after telling us a dirty, often sexist, joke. There were no women in our classes, and, of course, we all laughed at the jokes even if they weren't funny. After four months of this, I was shipped to a transfer company at Fort Dix, NJ, where we were supposed to "transfer" the troops returning from Europe. No troop ships came in during the next month, so I never found out what "transfer" meant. I was supposed to be stationed at Fort Dix for two months, but the army made a mistake and let me return home after one month. What I remember about my month at Fort Dix was playing pool with my first lieutenant, who was in the regular army, and serving on a court martial trial where some poor soul (who was guilty of being AWOL) had to go to prison in the stockade (I felt singularly unfitted to stand in judgment over him).

My First Job

My father said I would be working for him in the 60-bed nursing home we owned in the Bronx, the Hunts Point Home. My uncle had given it the following slogan, "A New Home for the Old." My father never told me actually what I was supposed to do in this "home." I was not replacing anybody, just being added to the administrative staff. I was supposed to check with Al Goll, the hospital administrator, across the street at the Hunts Point Hospital, as to precisely what my duties were to be. Unfortunately, Al didn't know either. An office was converted for me in a former storeroom in the basement of the nursing home. I had a small makeshift desk and a telephone. The nurse in charge, Ruth Schwartz, who ran the place, had an office on the first floor. Ruth cared about taking care of the patients. My responsibilities were minimal. I was to order the food. At first, I called two or three places to compare prices, but there seemed to be little difference. One heavily accented (from eastern Europe) salesman talked me into ordering the food only from him. The prices were the same, but since "I knew him" (I had never met him) the service would be "better." Of course, if I had any complaint, I could call him and the Home would get satisfaction.

I don't know where I got the idea (there wasn't much else to do), but I decided that part of my job was to visit patients, to learn how they liked the place, and to see how I could make things better for them without spending a great deal of money. On the first floor, there were nine private rooms. The second and third floors accommodated 20–25 patients each, in 2–4 bedded rooms. Very few of the patients could keep up their ends of a conversation. I remember one old man on the first floor, blind, with both legs amputated. He was always picking at himself, particularly his anus, and trying to get drunk on cough medicine. Another old lady was frightened of everything, and didn't want to be in the Home. Who could actually want to be there? The smell of urine was all too present. Many patients were permanently prone, or semipermanently tied into armchairs, or unable to talk. Visitors were few. Televisions blared continuously. The staff tried to take good care of the patients—feeding, washing, and combing them. The food was good; I ate it myself. The place was kept pretty clean. As my duties were minimal, I often took the subway down to my father's office where we discussed how to get patients for whom the City paid higher rates (but not about how to improve care at the home) and family affairs.

"A New Home for the Old"

The Hunts Point Home operated as a very simple organization. The day staff included a registered nurse and a licensed practical nurse, supplemented by several nurses aides, dietary, and housekeeping workers. Finances were handled by the hospital accounting staff across the street. Doctors paid very infrequent visits. Most of the payments for patients came from the city under the welfare program. Patients received custodial rather than rehabilitative care. Staff training was minimal. The staff was caring and the costs were low. As my father liked to say, these patients were receiving better care than they had been receiving before they came into the Home. He didn't say that care was comparable to that given in other facilities (I had no way of knowing this in any event). Of course, my job was superfluous. Presumably I was "learning the business." Although I honestly tried to learn about what was going on, I had no supervision other than conversations with the supervising nurse, the LPN, and the hospital administrator. I don't recall talking with my father in any detail about what was going on, and I don't recall him ever visiting the Home.

As the new Hunts Point Home administrator, I had to be interviewed and approved by the Inspections Department at the New York City Department of Hospitals. In response to questions about my youth and lack of experience, I replied that my authority was limited, I was learning on the job, and there was a qualified hospital administrator almost next door. During my tenure at the Home, the employees struck, seeking unionization; I recall thinking how unfair it was for employees to be marching outside carrying picket signs claiming that my father drove a Cadillac (when he, or rather his chauffeur, actually drove a Packard). Dad certainly didn't drive this car based on the profits he was making from the Home. I extinguished a fire caused by one of the employees, who threw a lighted cigar into a linen basket. The strike was brief, and the employees succeeded in becoming unionized. The leader of their union subsequently went to jail for stealing from his members. And then, life at the Home went on as before.

On Nursing Home Care

What I learned at the Hunts Point Home was the realities of for-profit care for the poor and elderly, and about the kindnesses of the hard-working, lowly paid, mostly black, employees in such an establishment. I learned about how difficult it was to take care of elderly, frail patients and why they seldom complained. One nurse who was accused of handling patients roughly was fired. I talked to the patients about her, but many were afraid to talk for fear of reprisals. I learned about how important food was to the old sick people. I learned about the callousness of families who had virtually thrown these people away, I learned that the patients wanted, more than anything else, someone to talk to, someone who would listen to them, and I prided myself that at least I forced myself to go upstairs to listen.

This kind of nursing home still exists, even as giant corporations have been formed with thousands and thousands of beds and patients. Medicaid is the major form of financing for nursing home care, which is plainly charity care for poor people. The corporations and homes are organized to make money from sick people, and frankly, unlike many of my colleagues, I have never seen anything wrong with this, since doctors, and nonprofit hospitals, and even professors of health policy and management, have always made money from sick people. But I wonder at the disproportionate share of the health care dollar that goes to acute medical care, and at the large number of Americans who lack health insurance coverage. It has long seemed to me that health care should be financed in some ways similar to education, where everyone is entitled and gets paid for 12 years of elementary and high school education. Similarly, I believe that everyone should be entitled to and get paid for hospital and nursing home care which is "medically" and "socially" necessary.

Learning Management From My Father

I learned a lot from my father. He taught me small things, such as how to fold an 8" by 10" piece of paper into a smaller envelope by first folding the paper in half and then into thirds. I always think of him now when doing such folding. He corrected my writing to "forty" on a check rather than "fourty." My father's word was his bond, which he never went back on, most particularly, with me. Dad said that the mark of a gentleman was being able to feel comfortable at the Waldorf Astoria as well as the Automat, presumably with the usual company that you would find in either place.

Dad keenly impressed upon me the difference between a dollar received or earned and a dollar kept from Uncle Sam.My father's idea of a good business was when you could put money in your pocket as the owner or entrepreneur, without actually coming to work. To put it in Marxian terms, he preferred to make money off the work of others. As a real estate speculator, he also believed in borrowing huge sums, the interest becoming a deductible business expense, and gambling on the financial health of the American economy (and the government's preference for paying back debt in inflated dollars) to earn large returns on small amounts of invested capital. He applied a similar approach to gambling on the stock market. My father insisted that although he was a gambler, he always knew how to limit his losses, which was the case so far as I knew.

What I learned about management from my father was the contrast in his behavior and performance to that of my flamboyant uncle. Uncle Harold was extremely smart and well-educated and was always talking, psychoanalyzing, and seducing women. My father, on the other hand was usually quiet (he dressed conservatively), and when he was angry he spoke in a very quiet (and to me menacing) voice. He listened to rather than talked at other people, never told them what to do, tried to work things out, and to be reasonable. He didn't care about being liked by everyone, but he always tried to do the right, reasonable thing, at least as he saw it. As a way to attract physicians to use our hospital, Dad tried to help them with their business, and with their personal lives, and to meet their demands as long as they were affordable. My uncle might curse out these same doctors as constipated know-nothings or as latent homosexuals, or as arrogant, greedy whiners and complainers.

Lessons Learned About Myself

Sad to say, I don't think I learned much about myself, working at the Hunts Point Home. My abnormal (in a statistical sense) upbringing, relative to my peers, has handicapped me as a manager, although not, I think, as a teacher of management. Simply, I was not brought up, as are most other children, in the frequent company of either parent, or in the company of children other than my brother. My upbringing failed to equip me with key social skills, and I valued intelligence and fashion to the detriment of mechanical or manual skills. Also, like many white upper middle-class men who grew up in the 1950s, I was ignorant of people from other cultural and socioeconomic backgrounds.

My father certainly did me a great disservice in telling me to go to school to have a good time, and then putting me to work for him. He may have done this as a result of his own youth. My father, second oldest of four, had been ignored by his own parents (his mother had died when he was a young man). Uncle Harold was the oldest child. My father played sports morning until night, until he was injured playing football, after which he told me he went out looking for fights. He studied business as an undergraduate, and saw an adult man's work as making a lot of money in the fastest way possible. The family had lost all their money through speculation in the Great Depression. Money impacted my father tremendously. He told me the story of eating with his in-laws when times were good and being complimented on his hearty appetite, and then after losing his money (his wife soon to go sailing to Europe with his mother-in-law) being told that he ate like a pig. My father had to look for work as a construction worker in the Depression. He had been through hard times, and he wanted me to be happy and have good times. I never talked to him about why he wanted me to work for him (although I knew he liked my company). We had talked about what I was going to do, and he didn't see the point in law school. "Aren't you going to work with me? You will always be well provided for," Dad used to say. This was good enough for me. I didn't know a lot of people my father's age who were doing different kinds of work, and no one encouraged me to do anything different.

Leaving the Home?

After 18 months, I wasn't learning anything new at the Hunts Point Home. I didn't have enough work to do. So, Dad suggested that I become his stockbroker (of course, he already had a stockbroker). This meant that I could kick back a good part of the commissions to him and learn something about the stock market. I had to take a course to learn how to be a registered representative and pass a test (also at the time, I took a course to learn how to pass the test to be an insurance salesman). Since I was a good student and test taker it was not difficult to pass the required exams. Then, I went to work as a registered representative, and actually learned something about the stock market. I even recruited some customers, most of whom were, of course, friends of my father's. What the job seemed to require was taking orders whether a customer wished to sell or buy 100 shares of U.S. Steel. I read up a lot about some individual companies, and visited one large corporation in which my father owned shares, General Tire in Akron, Ohio. There I talked with one of the owners who informed me about the company.

Early on, I figured out that my new job was no better than my first job, although the conditions of work, and the job location, were much nicer. And I reached the following conclusion on my own, that if eventually (I didn't see that day coming along soon) I was to take over the family business from my father and uncle, it would make sense that I should learn something about running their business. And so, I started to investigate graduate schools in hospital administration.

Graduate School

I was accepted by Cornell, where I had gone as an undergraduate (and where my brother was then an undergraduate). At Cornell, hospital administration was part of the Graduate School of Business and Public Administration (BPA). My memories of my graduate education are indistinct. I recall taking the introductory course in hospital administration from an ex-hospital administrator and thinking I could teach this course better myself. As an undergraduate, all the courses I had taken (except accounting and insurance) I had taken as part of a liberal education, as a preparation to be a "civilized person." These courses, obviously, had nothing to do with work. The two "useful" courses I had taken, in insurance and accounting, I found deathly boring, and had barely passed due to my lack of work. My lack of interest in such subjects continued in graduate school. To my classmates' amazement, I preferred courses in organizational theory: that is to say, how organizations were and should be structured and operated to the functional business courses such as finance and marketing. I found the theories interesting and Professor Rod White, a congenial professor. Most business school students found management, and particularly theory courses deadly dull, with these courses having the lowest prestige among the professorate, who clearly preferred finance and marketing.

Still in my library (and I throw out most of the books in my office which I haven't read recently) is a slim red volume by James G. March and Herbert A. Simon, *Organizations,* published in 1958. This book influenced me by making me think. Prior to graduate school, although I had worked in several organizations, I had never thought about why individuals work for a particular organization, why they continue to work for an organization, why they are motivated to work at their highest levels, or how they can be motivated to be more productive. March and Simon in chapter 4 argue that "the decision to participate lies at the core of the theory of 'organizational equilibrium,' the conditions of survival of an organization. Equilibrium reflects the organization's success in arranging payments to its participants adequate to motivate their continued participation."

A related concept is how an organization can structure incentives so that workers are motivated appropriately. Obviously, providing incentives has a cost and it is variously difficult to isolate the contribution of such incentives to an individual worker's performance. What fascinated me, and continues to fascinate me, is that those who manage the organization can consider and address questions like this, that certain systems of incentives in organizations work or don't work under different circumstances, and that presumably those who know more about structuring incentives can influence their organizations to operate better and be more successful, as compared to those who know less. An analogy can be drawn to coaches of sports teams who can more or less successfully channel the competitive efforts of their players.

In graduate school there was a continuing bias among the health care faculty against for-profit health care organizations, certainly strange at a program located within a business school. Indeed, Cornell B&PA eventually booted out the health and government programs and became strictly a graduate school of business. The health program had a notable guest lecturer, a former N.Y. state commissioner of health, who lectured against the evils of for-profit ownership in health care, and I remember standing up to him and defending the for-profits. (There weren't any chain hospital corporations at that time like Columbia-HCA.) My arguments went something like this: (1) as much variability exists among health care organizations under for-profit ownership as among organizations that are governmentally or nonprofit owned, so that very good for-profit and nonprofit organizations have more in common than nonprofits or for-profits do as a class; (2) physicians are largely engaged in for-profit health care, so for-profit hospitals are no worse than for-profit physicians; and, (3) capitalism is the American way of life, and for-profits are capitalist.

Reflection: Are For-Profits for You?

Many persons decide upon a career in nonprofits, or change careers to health care either because they want to do well by doing good, or because of a bad experience in working in a for-profit company with an excessive concern for profit and for nothing else. Consider these situations facing health care managers:

1. Sam Sparks works for a for-profit whose owner's main concern is to make money by doing things as cheaply as possible, and charging as much as possible.

2. Joy Jellinek works for a nonprofit whose top management's main concern is to keep their jobs and salaries high, and who generally want to do things as cheaply as possible, or to charge as much as possible.

3. Kyung-mi Kim enjoys working for herself in health care, selling her services to for-profit or not-for-profit health care organizations, doing quality work, and obtaining sufficient work to make a decent living.

I agree with Charles Handy (1998), who suggests that an increasing number of people who possess marketable sets of skills will be working for themselves as independent for-profit contractors. There's a wonderful feeling about being your own boss, even though (or especially) because this is for-profit. Can you think of a finer cause than feeding yourself and your dear ones? The difficulties are that independent contractors have to work longer hours and revenues come in large chunks and are uncertain.

Large nonprofits and large for-profits, are often not very different in practice. Of course, any profits in a for-profit go to owners and share-holders, while in nonprofits the board who acts as the owner cannot collect bonuses or dividends, and usually isn't paid. Yet the salaries for top managers and physicians in nonprofits are, I believe, overly high (over $500,000 for a chief executive of a mid-sized nonprofit hospital in New York City.)

In the case of smaller firms, (say from $5 to $50 million in revenues), however, the differences are probably greater. Nonprofits are driven and complicated by a sense of mission. This is why people work for them, give to them, and use them. Energy and leadership in service of mission is inspiring. As I have described above, complications follow when there is a lack of agreement as to what mission really means and regarding performance expectations among a variety of stakeholders.

For the last 20 years, I have worked for a university not-for-profit and on my own as a for-profit consulting firm (and as a for-profit author). While I was paying for my daughters to attend Princeton University, the revenues that I obtained for working from each of these two streams was roughly similar. Since their graduation, I have done less consulting, but I like the idea of getting paid according to what the market is willing to pay for my services. Such contracting focuses my attention.

Is For-Profit for You?: A Checklist

Yes   No

_____ _____ Do you think there is something definitely wrong with for-profit health care?

_____ _____ How comfortable are you with assuming risk, in your own business?

_____ _____ How important is it for you to work in an organization with a strong sense of mission?

_____ _____ How frustrated do you become in working for a nonprofit organization in which there is disagreement over goals and strategies?

_____ _____ Have you ever talked with managers in both for-profits and nonprofits and asked them to comment on what they think are the principal differences?

_____ _____ If all organizations in health care could only be either governmental, nonprofit or for-profit, do you think for-profit is best?

_____ _____ In assessing differences in performance of health care organizations, do you think auspice is a primary differentiating causal factor? Why?

_____ _____ Do you think large nonprofits should publicly disclose how they do business, in the same ways that for-profits do?

Practical Exercise

What organizations and managers do you particularly admire and why? Are they in the public, nonprofit, or for-profit sector? Interview managers in different sectors whose jobs are at similar levels, ask them what they like and don't like about their positions and why. Tell them you are considering obtaining a job like theirs some day, and ask their advice as to whether this is a good idea (would they do this again?). Ask them how you can obtain such a job, and whether it makes any difference to work in such a job in the public, nonprofit, or for-profit sector.

3

Managing Health Care for the Poor

A great deal happened between graduating from Cornell's Graduate School of B&PA in 1963, and my taking the job of associate administrator in 1967 at the Gouverneur Health Services program on New York City's lower East side. First, I got married. Second, my father died. Third, I saw that there was no place nor reason to work for my uncle and his new partner, his third wife, Rose, in the hospital business. Fourth, one of my professors, Rod White, suggested that since I was a good student, I should consider going for my doctorate, at government expense. He urged me to see Dr. Cecil Sheps at the Graduate School of Public Health at the University of Pittsburgh, which I did.

To make a long story short, I moved to Pittsburgh to pursue a Ph.D. in the Graduate School of Public and International Affairs (GSPIA) rather than in Public Health or in Sociology, two of the alternatives. My then wife, Marie-Claire, got a job working as a secretary for two internists, and I got a part-time job helping to write a newspaper for the United Mineworkers, a position which I subsequently quit because it took too much time away from my studies. I majored at GSPIA in Economic and Social Development and minored in Health Services Management at the Graduate School of Public Health. The chair of my doctoral committee was Charles Perrow, a noted organizational theorist, author of *Complex Organizations,* and subsequently of the fascinating book *Normal Accidents,* which explained why accidents, such as boats colliding at sea or Three Mile Island, are likely to and do happen. Perrow subsequently went to Yale. I wrote my dissertation under his supervision, applying his theories of the impact of technology of work on organizational structure in business organizations to nursing units in hospitals. I argued that nursing technology differs significantly among hospital nursing units but that nurse staffing doesn't adequately take this into account. Thus, there was considerable waste of skilled nursing resources in the more routine units, while in the more nonroutine units, nonprofessional nurses often did nonroutine work, for which they weren't adequately trained, because of the insufficient number of professional nurses. The study had a great advantage, for my subsequent management career, in my spending several weeks observing nursing and hospital work in eight nursing units in four hospitals. I also learned how to construct questionnaires and evaluate data.

Near the end of my studies, Dr. Sheps left the University of Pittsburgh to become general director of the Beth Israel Medical Center, a large academic medical center in New York City. I followed him to New York City, where he hired me as an assistant director, much in the way that my father had hired me at the nursing home. No one held this job before I assumed it, and I supervised two tiny departments, purchasing and the storeroom, in addition to doing undefined staff work, such as making a study of the efficiency of operating room scheduling for Dr. Sheps.

But after only a few months working at Beth Israel, a management turnover occurred in the large Gouverneur Ambulatory Care Program (GACU) which Beth Israel managed under contract with the City of New York. The administrator, Dr. Howard Brown, left to become head of New York City's Health and Hospitals Corporation, and the associate administrator, Harold Light, left to take a top management job at St. Vincent's Hospital. Dr. Sheps asked me to replace Light as associate director of the Gouverneur program while he was recruiting for Dr. Brown's successor. And so, without really knowing what I was getting into, I accepted the position. I thus started what was to be the most difficult job of my life, which I held for about three and one half years.

The Lower East Side

What is today one of the trendiest neighborhoods in New York was until very recently the first home for many European immigrants to the U.S. The neighborhood was home to a diverse mixture of ethnic groups—including, originally, all four of my grandparents who had for over 100 years lived in tenement housing. While many of these tenements had been replaced by once-new public housing, a large number of Gouverneur's clients (mostly old-time residents but also recent Puerto Rican and Chinese immigrants) continued to live in tenement housing. With few or no occupational skills and little command of English, many immigrants had difficulties with what seem to be the simplest processes of life—finding a place to live, a job, and providing for their children. Additionally, many suffered from parasitic disease, tuberculosis, narcotics addiction, dental disease, and other illnesses prevalent in low-income populations.

In the lower East side, Gouverneur served a population of about 126,000—comprised of approximately 42% Caucasian, 32% Puerto Rican, 18% Chinese, and 8% African American. Gouverneur's clients, however, were 18% Caucasian, 71% Puerto Ricans, 5% Chinese, and 6% African American. The difference in use of services among groups living in the area is explained in part by relation to place of residence and availability of public transportation, and also by the impact of cultural factors on access to health care.

The Gouverneur Health Services Program

Gouverneur functioned as a neighborhood health center some years before this concept was further developed and adopted nationally by the Office of Economic Opportunity in Washington, DC. In 1968, about 39,000 patients made 196,000 physician visits to the Gouverneur Ambulatory Care Unit (GACU), and to the Judson Health Center, a satellite center. Gouverneur had a full-time equivalent staff of about 350 employees, of whom almost one-sixth were salaried physicians.

Most services were provided at GACU, which was an old six-story brick building that bordered the East River Drive. This was an extremely crowded and noisy building. My office at first was on the fourth floor, next to the dental department. My introduction to an atmosphere of constant crises began immediately when the finance officer resigned and I realized the purchasing officer seldom appeared. Physician specialists and part-timers often didn't show as well, disappointing patients and making scheduling problematic. Behavioral health staff of psychiatrists and social workers didn't see eye to eye with many of the internists and pediatricians, and there were also conflicts between the director of nursing and the chiefs of Medicine and of Pediatrics. Governeur's staff was frequently in conflict with Beth Israel Hospital's, regarding, for example, the perceived quality of laboratory services. Gouverneur staff also argued with those purporting to represent the community, who wanted more jobs and power for themselves and their friends.

The previous administration had accomplished wonders, receiving national publicity and praise, and the previous administrators went on to higher positions elsewhere. (Dr. Howard Brown, the director, taught at NYU's Graduate School of Public Administration and was director of the health program before his untimely death, and Harold Light, the associate director, went on to become CEO of Long Island College Hospital.) Brown and Light operated Gouverneur according to 25 basic principles, which I think are of more than historical interest, in delivering health care to a low-income, diverse population. The principles raise as many questions as they answer, and perhaps this was one of their strengths. For examples, starting with principle number 1, how does an organization trade off between gearing services primarily to meet the needs of patients relative to meeting staff needs so that staff can be empowered to better serve patients? Practically speaking, what percent of budget should be spent on staff training, when patients' service needs are more or less unlimited?

Basic Principles: Gouverneur Health Services Program, 1967

1. The services belong to the patients and therefore should be geared primarily to meet their needs rather than those of the staff.

2. The services the patients are to receive are services to which they are entitled by right rather than by privilege and, therefore, are to be delivered in a manner which is conducive to meeting the patient's psychological, social, and emotional needs, as well as his biological ones.

3. The patient functions as part of a larger milieu—in his own home and in the broader community—and these forces, therefore, must be taken into account if the service rendered is to be meaningful.

4. The community at large is entitled to a voice in the program and should share in the decision-making process wherever possible.

5. The staff's activity, if it is to be meaningful, cannot be confined to the functioning within the four walls of the Gouverneur structure.

6. Professions other than medicine have significant contributions to make to the philosophical base of the institution and functional aspects of the program, and these views should be formally represented on a policy-making board similar to the medical board in a hospital.

7. Every effort is made to make the physical facility an attractive one to which patients come without revulsion, and creature comforts of the patients are reasonably catered to.

8. Lack of facility in English should not be a deterrent to communication with the staff, and toward this end as many multilingual neighborhood people as possible are employed to further the patient's sense of familiarity and comfort.

9. The service is made accessible, from a geographical and time standpoint to the degree that financing allows.

10. The traditional clinical subspecialties, which treat body organs rather than individuals, are eliminated or reduced to the lowest possible number.

11. Patients are seen, with the exception of care for acute needs, through a staggered appointment system.

12. The notion that lines were inevitable in clinics is not to be tolerated and every effort is to be made to keep lines from forming or people from standing while waiting for a particular service.

13. As many full-time or half-time physicians as possible are to be hired so that patients can return to the same doctor and identify with him as their family physician.

14. Full-time staff have no outside practice and all staff are to be paid for service at the clinic so that the tendency toward primacy of interest in fee-for-service practice might be eliminated, or reduced to the barest possible minimum.

15. The notion that one's work is done when one saw his last patient is not to be tolerated since this inevitably leads to collusion between doctors and nurses to "run patients through" with an eye toward going home early.

16. All professionals are paid for time—not just for services rendered—and consequently are expected to work the hours agreed upon prior to employment.

17. One's status as an employee does not entitle him to subject a patient to any indignity or scorn or derision and reports of such behavior are severely dealt with irrespective of the station of the employee involved.

18. Patients have, at all times, access to the administrator so that they may voice their views on the service rendered or the individual rendering the service, and every such report is checked out.

19. The administrative organization remains as loosely structured as feasible to reduce to the barest possible minimum the amount of flexibility which might be lost through bureaucratization.

20. The administrative structure is as "horizontal" as possible with both responsibility and authority pushed down to the level of least training which can perform the function required efficiently and economically.

21. Experimentation with new systems of care and administrative organization are encouraged to reduce costs while increasing efficiency.

22. Experimentation in new uses of personnel and the creation of new jobs for neighborhood people are encouraged both as a socially desirable goal and as a means of stretching health manpower.

23. All staff are encouraged to be innovative and to exercise as much initiative as they can muster in the interest of improving patient care.

24. The clinic facility is a vehicle for meeting patient needs and as such has no fixed territorial claims made upon it by staff or service seeking status or prestige in maintaining given offices or locations.

25. The clinic facility belongs to the community and as such is made available to the community for meetings and so forth, provided these do not conflict with patient care (Brown & Light, 1967).

Part of the reason I was selected for the job of Associate Director was to help "integrate" this neighborhood health center with the Beth Israel Hospital, about two miles away. What this meant was increased standardization, more organized referrals, and more conformance with uptown administrative policies. This system alignment, of course, was what the long-time neighborhood health center's professional leadership had been organized to fight against (see operating principles 19 and 20 above, which were certainly not followed at Beth Israel Hospital).

Gouverneur's 25 basic operating principles seem remarkable to me even now. And they were mostly followed and carried out before and, for several years, after I worked there.[1] The principles represent a version of many of the aspects of self-managing teams and network organizations, trumpeted by Tom Peters (1987), among others, as the only and the best way to manage in today's competitive markets. These basic operating principles were implemented to provide services to the poor and unenfranchised, many of whom were foreigners. In contrast to the clients, most of the professional staff at GACU were white and middle class, and indeed most of the funds to provide service were provided by white, working class taxpayers.

New leadership was successful in temporarily transforming service delivery at GACU in large part because of the scandals involving the old Gouverneur Hospital, which had lost both its hospital and teaching accreditations by 1961. It was recommended then that the hospital be closed. But the community and its advocates—including a number of well-organized, voluntary social agencies, influenced the city of New York to contract with the Beth Israel Hospital to provide personal and emergency services to ambulatory patients in the old facility. Dr. Brown and Mr. Light were able to organize the community behind the reforms

---

[1] At the time of my last visit, in 1995, however, I observed that Gouverneur was violating all the above basic operating principles. It had become a typical large city outpatient clinic operated by the New York City Health and Hospitals Corporation. Ironically, the City is, in 1998, supposedly beginning to attempt to transform—i.e. reinvent at least some of the 25 principles, in the face of losing patients to managed care.

they wished to carry out and then to attract professional physicians and nurses to provide the new model of care.

Organizational Structure and Management

Gouverneur had six main service units: Medicine, Pediatrics, an experimental Family Health Unit, OB-GYN, Dental, and Emergency. Supporting services included lab, x-ray, pharmacy, medical records, housekeeping and building maintenance, security, purchasing, finance, and personnel. GACU also ran an ambulance service, and a satellite health center in the western part of our service area. The health center was open Saturday and had evening hours, four evenings a week.

Gouverneur should have been an impossible place to run for many reasons, and yet it ran as well as it did, for a fairly long time, because of the enthusiasm and dedication of its staff. Two examples demonstrate some of the management challenges at Gouverneur: the family health unit (FHU), and the financial and accounting function. Most of the best professionals in the organization had pioneered in developing a family health unit. The theory behind the unit was to organize a team of providers to serve a geographical subarea. The unit included a heavy dose of psychiatrists, psychologists, social workers, and social health technicians because behavioral problems represented a large part of the population's health problems. Extending the FHU concept was problematic, however. Three main issues existed: (1) conflict over which staff disciplines should be included; (2) disagreement about the feasibility of attracting full-time FHU staff to work in the unit; and (3) differences on the desirability of including existing patients of FHU physicians, who lived in other geographic areas in any particular FHU. For example, pediatricians were included as part of the FHU team although the chief of Pediatrics was against the concept (he argued that children would be better taken care of when treated by a specialized staff in a waiting area only for children); obstetricians did not want to be included despite the preferences of the FHU leadership; dentists wanted to be part of the unit but could not be physically accommodated because of equipment costs and staffing. Moreover, all the physician staff in the FHUs were not full-time or half-time (it was difficult to recruit such physicians); the pilot FHU was accused of obtaining more than their fair share of support services, relative to the other Medicine and Pediatrics units. Most importantly, the pilot FHU started by taking in all existing patients of the physicians working in the unit. These patients resided throughout the whole catchment area, rather than only in one small geographic area; and, patient records were kept only for individuals, for legal and other reasons, rather than for families. The FHU leadership wanted to relate each FHU to a specific neighborhood, and to convert the entire facility into six FHUs. Most of the GACU staff was opposed or indifferent.

I had the good fortune, at this time, to be working with Marv Rosenberg, a community organizer, whom I promoted to assistant director. His efforts were essential in the implementation of the new structure. Marv was convinced that the new structure would work better than the old. He believed that we had to extend the concept or disband the pilot FHU, in which the GACU clinical leadership was situated and many of whom might leave. Marv believed the changes to be necessary—such as converting the record system to family records and forcing many families to change regular providers, even as their implementation required a great deal of time and effort. The new structure would result in better service to families, not only because of family needs for social services, but also because many of our patient families were headed by young parents with many children who would benefit by being seen together by the same staff. Most of my reservations about the new structure were with regard to feasibility and cost of the required new physical construction and relocation. Marv's willingness to take full responsibility for implementation, coupled with his infectious enthusiasm and the trust he generated among staff convinced me in favor of conversion to FHUs.

The FHU conversion was never subjected to a rigorous evaluation, nor was the matrix management[2] scheme I implemented to go along with it. Again, this was a wonderful idea in theory which didn't exactly pan out in practice. It failed not because the theory was wrong, among other reasons, but because it was difficult to recruit and keep talented staff at Gouverneur. My own admittedly informal evaluation (views which I still retain) was that the new system worked better than the old system, and that with a suitable front end investment, we could have made the whole system work and work much better for patients.

For me, the other interesting management structure challenge was relations between the neighborhood health center and the hospital. In a case history about the situation written in 1969 (Kovner, Kahane, Katz, & Sheps, 1969), I, together with colleagues, argued the benefits of a

---

[2] Matrix management involved all nurses in the FHUs reporting in a *line* relationship to the team leaders and a staff advisory relationship to nursing (similarly with clerical staff). The concept was one boss (team leader) for clinical service and another (professional chief) for staff development and professional standards within the occupations.

formally structured relationship. Such a relationship was beneficial to the neighborhood health center for the following reasons: higher priority for Gouverneur patients referred for specialty and inpatient care at the hospital; (2) staff privileges for Gouverneur physicians at the hospital; (3) increased ability, because of the opportunities through affiliation with Beth Israel for adequate professional career development, to recruit and keep high quality staff; and (4) access for Gouverneur to skilled services of hospital administrative and technical staff. The hospital also benefitted from such a relationship in the following ways: (1) the broadening of the scope of services provided its own patients and community, which would then include provision of home care and medical services to nursing home patients; (2) a more welcoming attitude toward low-income women delivering in the hospital who had not received prenatal care at the hospital, and establishment of evening and appointment services for all clinic patients; (3) the influencing of physician training programs to be more concerned with the whole patient rather than merely the patient's disease, and (4) facilitating admission of Gouverneur patients to the hospital.

Of course, reality was a bit different from the article we wrote. Five major problems challenged Gouverneur clinical management: (1) numerous glitches regarding "hand-offs" to the hospital and back to the health center concerning services to and information about Gouverneur patients; (2) Gouverneur staff didn't think the Medical Center outpatient services should be organized as a clinic or that services provided to Gouverneur patients be "clinic" services; (3) Dr. Sheps hired a new GACU physician director, but the two did not get along well, the physician director being acutely dissatisfied with his pay and benefits as well as with the status of the Gouverneur physicians within the hospital medical hierarchy; (4) I was severely constrained in hiring a competent controller because of hospital pay scales, and when, with the hospital's help, I was able to recruit a controller, he spent a good part of his time, unfortunately, on site at the hospital rather than giving me the management data that I needed. The Beth Israel controller was constantly trying to maximize Gouverneur overhead contribution from third parties to the hospital; and (5) many of us thought that Beth Israel medical staff saw Gouverneur as second class and providing charity care.

Lessons Learned About Health Care Delivery

First I finally had a real management job as day-to-day administrator. Gouverneur was operating better, I believe, because of my interventions. I was successful in the job because I was intelligent, worked hard, and had a firm belief in the basic principles of the previous Gouverneur leadership. I also attached the greatest importance to quality of care and service. I held to these principles because I saw what impact they had on the delivery of care and that this resulted in happier professionals (most of them) and healthier patients (some of them). For my personal development, I gained increasing familiarity with a diverse clientele, many of whom were more interested in getting adequate jobs than in obtaining adequate health care. I also learned about the importance of behavioral and environmental health, and the difficulties of launching cooperative programs integrating ambulatory health services with the city health department.

Lessons Learned About Management at Gouverneur

Most importantly, through my position at Gouverneur, I gained confidence in myself. This new confidence was of great significance to me, given my previous lack of work experience. In addition to supporting clinic operations, I was fully engaged in contract negotiations with the city, the state and even the federal government through the Office of Economic Opportunity. I also began, with Dr. Sheps' help, to examine and write up my experiences. Such reflection has proved to be invaluable for me in understanding how organizations function and helping me focus on how to further improve organizational and individual performance.

My experience at Gouverneur validates the theory concerning the lag between technological innovation and structural change. Making structural change is commonly very costly—building a new structure from scratch is politically much easier than converting an old structure in an existing facility. It is much easier to recruit staff who participate because they want to work in a new structure rather than to convert existing professionals who have had success in practice and who were successfully trained in a different way of doing things.

At Gouverneur, I had my first experience firing employees. The most important lesson I learned was that, generally, ineffective people are fired too late, if at all. In my view, if inadequate people are not fired after 18 months, then their presence becomes as much the organization's fault as the individual's. The first person I fired was a department head who had a terrible attendance record. He explained to me that he was sick, and had personal problems. I gave him more slack than I should have. Subsequently, after he had been fired, I discovered that he was an inveterate gambler, who had borrowed money from numerous employees, including some who worked for him, and was deeply in debt.

The second person I fired was Will Jonas, a finance person whom I myself had hired because he was the least bad alternative available. The first sign of trouble was the lateness of the monthly statement that I had instituted and required. (This was important relative to hiring the right numbers of employees for the right numbers of hours as related to governmentally approved grant budgets.) At this point, I spoke to Will after discovering that what he finally submitted was full of mistakes. Next I began to hear complaints concerning his rudeness, arrogance, and insensitivity to the poor whom he called "welfare chiselers." In addition, Will told me that he had to report late twice a week because he had to see a psychiatrist and that he would stay later, but I never found him around after regular working hours. I kept Will on for over 6 months. The controller at the hospital, to whom Will also reported, was satisfied with Will's work and said that Gouverneur was in good financial shape and there was nothing to worry about. The GACU physician executive director (my boss) told me to do what I wanted to do, since the hospital controller was not opposed to my doing so.

At that time, New York state passed a regulation that required all possible efforts to collect fees from those who could pay before city agencies could receive reimbursement from Medicaid. Will's attitude toward this directive forced me to fire him. When it came to implementing the collections, Will demanded that the registration staff who were to collect the money be part of his department or that a separate cashier's office be set up on the first floor of the facility. Marv Rosenberg, however, argued that the registration staff should continue as part of the family health units because of their other duties, the lack of available space on the first floor for a cashier's office, and because it was not fair to patients to make them stand in two lines before seeing a health professional. I sided with Marv and instructed Will to develop an implementation plan under which he would be responsible for the cash collection aspects of the registrar's work. After two weeks, he had not devised the plan, and so, I fired him. Although Will's subordinates were able to do his routine work in the accounting department, I was still never to get the management data categorized and with the variances that I had wanted.

Did I deal with Will appropriately? I have taught the case at NYU, calling it, "The Associate Director and the Controllers" (Kovner, 1980). Most of my students agree that I should have fired Will. A substantial number of each year's class, however, say that I should have spent more time with Will up front explaining what I wanted and helping him learn how to give me what I required. At that time, however, I felt that I didn't have the time to do so, and was not a trained accountant. In hindsight, I feel I should have spent more time personally recruiting someone who met or could meet my specifications, and who shared Gouverneur's values. I had relied on the hospital's personnel department for recruiting, but I should have done the recruiting myself, spending as much time as it took until I had landed a more suitable candidate.

The experience highlights the importance of the fit between the skills and experience a job candidate possesses and the requirements of the job itself. Will might have succeeded as an assistant hospital controller, while he failed at Gouverneur. Also, despite infinite pains some managers may take, they will not always recruit the successful candidate. (This does imply a longer and more intensive recruiting process). Recruiting failures usually occur because one or both sides weren't honest enough up front, because either side lacked an adequate conception of what was really required to do the job successfully.

Why Did I Leave Gouverneur?

After two years, the physician executive director of Gouverneur left for an administrative job in a hospital upstate. He was replaced by another physician director, Dr. Flux, from the Bronx. Both of these individuals were M.D.s with administrative experience in large ambulatory care programs like Gouverneur's. At the time, however, I failed to see the value that they added to our organization other than that they were necessary buffers between medical administration at the hospital and at Gouverneur. Then Dr. Sheps, himself, left to become vice president for medical affairs at the University of North Carolina.

Dr. Sheps' replacement was a renowned physician executive, Dr. Ray Trussell, who had been commissioner of the Health and Hospitals Corporation and who had developed and implemented the city's vast affiliation program between the municipal hospitals and academic medical centers. Dr. Trussell visited Gouverneur and told us of all the good things that he would do for us and for our partnership. I don't recall what it was that I said, but I questioned him in front of the staff whether something that he said was true or was it really possible to do as he said in such a short time. Dr. Trussell, naturally, did not appreciate my questions, and refused to work with me. Thus my time at Gouverneur ended abruptly, and I had to find a new job.

Relating to New Management

I have heard both sides on the issue of speaking the truth to power. Some say they want to work for a boss to whom they can speak up while they in turn are supportive to subordinates. Others say that what works is managerial subservience to a boss and harshness with subordinates. I'm sure it can work either way, or somewhere in between, for example, speaking your mind more through indirection, asking the boss leading questions or supplying him with data and letting the boss draw his own conclusions. In my case, I was unaware that Trussell (rather than Flux) was really my boss, and that as such, he expected a certain deference from me. Whether the manager chooses to speak his or her mind or not is the manager's choice. I recommend, however, that managers consider the price they may have to pay for saying to the boss what is on their minds.

Reflection: Learning About Diversity

As I reflect on the Gouverneur experience, I see this more as a learning experience in working with diversity. How one feels about diversity depends on one's own demographic characteristics and history. However, as a manager in 2000, this is an issue that you will have to deal with. I see "diversity" more as an issue of human development where every one gets a chance and everyone has special needs and special interests. Obviously, this plays out differently in the United States over the last 40 years. Consider the following situations facing heath care managers:

1. Tony Biles, a White male, complains that he has not been promoted to the position he has interviewed for, which is offered instead to a Latino female whom he thinks lacks his qualifications.
2. Tyrone Sharps is the token Black employee in a large ambulatory care center in a close-in suburban area. He feels that the other management and clinical employees who are predominantly White (male or female) do not invite him to social events nor does he get, as others do, all the information important for him to properly do his job.
3. Marie Fong, from Taiwan, insists that she is being offered jobs only in clinics serving Asian populations (including Koreans) rather than in "mainstream" HMOs whose managers are primarily white. At one interview, someone tells her that "you should try and get a job at the public hospital because you don't fit in here."

All of us belong to some minority group. All of us don't fit in as well as we might in certain groups in certain organizations. For example, my parents were Jewish and I remember being called " kike" riding in a bus in Baltimore as a teenager. I have heard many derogatory comments about Jews in work situations. Discrimination does not apply only to cultural or religious characteristics. I have been told repeatedly that I was overqualified because of my PhD when applying for management jobs. I know that persons have felt uncomfortable working with me, as a manager, because of my "superior" education. I am not saying that all people are to the same extent systematically discriminated against because of one of the demographic groups that we belong to. Yet, it is important to understand what groups others recognize us as belonging to, and what that signifies for them.

There is a "downside" to being a White, male, heterosexual manager, as there is to managing as a member of any minority group. Everyone is prejudiced against strangers and likes people whom they see in important ways as similar to themselves. This may be in terms of values rather than demographic characteristics. And people don't always say what they mean or behave as they say. White, male, heterosexual managers often ask themselves "What do women, gays, and people of color want? What should they want?" Women, gays, and people of color who are managers, ask themselves, "When push comes to shove, can I really trust white, heterosexual males to give us an even break? Given past history, we deserve at least an even break, maybe more than an even break, other things being equal."

Leaving aside questions of equal opportunity and affirmative action (I don't feel I have anything distinctive to say about these matters), it is important for managers to think before speaking ("how are members of different groups going to react to what I want to say?") and to listen when others speak to hear what they aren't saying (for example, does this mean that I, and members of my group are included in that generalization, policy, or procedure?). If you, as manager, do make a mistake, at least make every effort to do things very right the next time or regarding a "recovery." The easiest way not to make a mistake, of course, is to think before speaking, and to consider how members of different groups might react, having made some effort, in advance, to learn about relevant differences and perceptions among groups commonly encountered in your workplace.

I believe in equal opportunity, and in reaching out to assure equal opportunity to minority groups. I do not believe in hiring and promoting people because they are members of minority groups when they are less qualified than other candidates for specific positions. Of course "less qualified" can often not be scientifically determined, at least to the satisfaction of all involved. For many positions there is a distinct advantage to the organization in hiring and promoting minority candidates, for example, in jobs which involve considerable interface and trust-building with minority communities.

Learning About Diversity

Yes   No

_____ _____ Do you think that managers of certain minority groups perform better or worse than their white, male, heterosexual counterparts?

_____ _____ Do you know how managers in your organization are viewed by staff who are members of minority groups?

_____ _____ Do you know how members of minority groups, as employees and as customers, are viewed by front-line workers and persons in positions of power in your organization?

_____ _____ Do you have a good understanding of the cultures of minority groups as employees and customers, as this affects your work?

_____ _____ Do you think that members of other minority groups at work feel they have any equal chance, as you do, to be employed and promoted?

_____ _____ Do you think they have the same chance of getting what they want as you do? (Why or why not?)

_____ _____ Is it important to you to work in a health care organization in which diversity is importantly valued? (Why or why not?)

Practical Exercise

Consider what it would be like to work in an organizaton where most of the people at the manager's level are members of groups other than those to which the manager belongs. For example, if the manager is a White, heterosexual male, imagine working for a large health care organization whose top managers are all nonheterosexual women of color. Would you, as a manager, be forced to behave any differently in such an organization? Does the manager imagine that persons who belong to groups other than those you belong behave any differently toward the manager because of their minority status? Interview managers who belong to ethnic and gender groups different than your own and ask them to share experiences and give you advice about experiencing and managing diversity.

4

Managing in Academia

I went to the University of Pennsylvania in 1970 because I couldn't find a job in New York. I had a second job opportunity in Philadelphia, with the Albert Einstein Medical Center, in north Philadelphia, as an assistant administrator with the mercurial Bob Sigmond, CEO (whom I was to work with subsequently at New York University, and who had been on the faculty at the University of Pittsburgh when I had been pursuing my doctoral degree at the Graduate School of Public and International Affairs there in 1963). The job I accepted was as group practice administrator for the Department of Medicine at the University of Pennsylvania.

Again, the position didn't exist prior to my occupying it. I was recruited by Bill Kissick, the ebullient chair of the Department of Community Medicine, who also had a faculty appointment in the Wharton School of Business, which was just across Spruce Street. My principal responsibilities were to bring management expertise to the outpatient clinics and to the newly formed group practice, both of which had been operating without an administrator. I received a faculty appointment in Community Medicine and eventually in the Management Department of the Wharton School where I would be involved in starting the new graduate program in health care administration, being planned by Dr. Kissick, and by Professor Robert Eilers, an economist in Wharton's Insurance Department.

My boss at the medical school was to be Arnold "Bud" Relman, later editor of the New England Journal of Medicine, who was chair of the Department of Medicine. Relman's deputy director was Dr. Samuel Thier, later to become president of Brandeis University and then president and CEO of Partners Health System, a merger of the Massachusetts

General Hospital and the Brigham Hospitals, and a former fraternity brother of mine at Cornell.

When I first arrived in Philadelphia, I felt as I had in the cellar of my father's nursing home in the Bronx. Now that I was there, what was I really to do? My first step was to talk to everyone relevant to my potential contribution. First there was Dr. Relman. Although he claimed to want to bring management to development of the group and use of the clinics, he was principally interested in medical research and teaching. And he was very busy. I soon discovered that a principal problem for physicians was the amounts and distribution of revenues. During an orientation period I learned that many of the physicians in private practice were unhappy with Dr. Relman's plans to include all practice income as part of the department rather than continuing as solo fee-for-service practitioners (although existing practice was to be grandfathered in). Physicians who were salaried and saw private patients in the group practice had been recruited to the Department of Medicine primarily to do research and teaching. There was no half-time or full-time physician "in charge" of the group practice. Was this what I was supposed to manage?

Another problem was how space in the outpatient clinics was terribly underutilized and continuity of care was low. Although I wrote a report on how to better use the space, it was never implemented as this didn't fit with clinician and resident schedules. The situation reminded me of a similar report I had submitted at Beth Israel Hospital, prior to taking the job at Gouverneur, making recommendations to improve productivity in the use of the operating rooms, similarly never implemented because operating surgeons, those with preferred schedules, didn't see it as in their interest to change. The lesson to be learned from this is that significant change will not be implemented unless the powers that be see this change as being in *their* interest.

At the University of Pennsylvania, similarly to my experience at Beth Israel, I had been recruited in part because of my vita and connections. There was a feeling at first that eventually there would be a use for me, if the precise job to which I had been recruited didn't work out, or could be handled by someone with less impressive credentials. After about a year in my job, I was recruited away by the Wharton School to be the first director of the graduate program in health care administration. That first year remains in part a blur to me, mainly because of personal problems including a sudden divorce.

Back at the university, I kept two jobs for a while, but before long my heart and soul was busy working for Dr. Eilers, a professor of Insurance at the Wharton School. I was chosen to direct the new program, primarily because the first director-to-be, Howard Newman (subsequently to be my dean at N.Y.U.), had become director of the Health Care Financing Administration (HCFA) in Washington, D.C. Bob Eilers had learned to trust me and appreciate my skills and experience in helping to accomplish his agenda, which was to form a first-class department of health care administration, almost from scratch, in a first-class school of business.

Who Was Bob Eilers?

When I knew him 25 years ago, Bob Eilers was about 40 years old, tall, thin, with large hands and a friendly smile. A full professor at the Wharton School, his PhD was in economics, and his academic interest was health care insurance. His dreams were large. Bob was originally from Iowa. He attended Drake University, and worked at the University of Pennsylvania most of his professional life. He was a commander in the Navy, an elder in the Lutheran Church, and he had built his own house in the country in Northeastern Pennsylvania. At ease with insurance moguls, he was sometimes uncomfortable with the posturing of academics. Bob was the best boss I ever had.

Bob was an ideal boss for the following reasons: He never told me how to do what he expected me to do, but rather listened to what I had to say. He asked me leading questions, and usually did not interrupt. He got me the staff, space, and travel funds that I needed to do the job. He took an interest in my academic career, read all my papers, and gave me the most helpful criticism (although we were in different fields). He sat in on my classes and helped me become a better teacher. He also took an interest in my personal life and was a dear friend, as was his wife, Delores, to me and my new wife, Chris.

Perhaps some of the reason for his success was due to his hard work and rather unusual workday. Usually, he worked nine to five, like everyone else. Next, he went home to dinner with his family. Then, at about 9 PM he put in a second workday, usually until 2 AM. After 5 hours of sleep, he was ready for the next day.

Bob raised the money for the new program in health care administration. The fund included capital to redesign an existing building, for which he oversaw massive renovations. The insurance department occupied one floor in our building, the health care faculty, another floor, and the top and bottom floors were devoted to classrooms and meeting rooms. Our strategy was to recruit young faculty in other departments and buy part of their salary, fund their research, and involve them in consulting.

Bob Eilers' Views on National Health Insurance

Bob's approach has keyed my thinking on this important subject, and his ability to articulate a leadership view on the major health policy issue of the time also motivated me in working with him. I will focus my discussion on an article Bob wrote in two parts for *The New England Journal of Medicine* on April 22 and 29, 1971, 28 years ago. The special article is entitled "National Health Insurance: What Kind and How Much." The *NEJM* abstract reads as follows:

The major forces behind the movement for national health insurance— health care costs, suboptimal mortality and morbidity levels, dissatisfaction with health care delivery and limitations of private insurance—must be considered in the development of criteria for evaluating national health insurance proposals. Although financial accessibility for health care for all citizens is a necessary criterion, the acceptability of all health care delivery arrangements to individual consumers is of equal importance. A reorientation of health delivery, emphasizing efficiency by imposing upon physicians both financial accountability opportunities to share in cost savings, is a vital ingredient for any proposal. Also, to be acceptable, a proposal must articulate a comprehensive plan for phasing in the program over a period of possibly a decade. Other objectives are minimization of governmental regulation, consumer participation in cost, and maintenance of quality of care.

He began by describing the problems in the current system: namely, high costs, the comparatively unfavorable levels of mortality and morbidity, dissatisfaction with health delivery, and the limitations of private health insurance. He next presented his criteria for evaluating national health insurance proposals: financial accessibility, delivery acceptability, cost efficiency, phased implementation, minimization of governmental regulation, consumer participation in cost, and quality of care.

Then, he examined current proposals for national health insurance, and generically categorized them into three groups: (a) voluntary or mandatory purchase by the bulk of the population of private health insurance with basic health benefits, with modest deductibles, if any; (b) catastrophic coverage plans; and, (c) a national health system with centralized control of both the financing and delivery arrangements by the federal government. He criticized all proposals for either considering little or no change in delivery arrangements or mandating specific delivery arrangements.

Bob presented his own desired vision of competition among large health care organizations under national health insurance. He acknowledged the limitations of (skills and experience) among organized purchasers, but believed this would evolve. He recommended that Medicare remain largely unchanged with Medicaid federally financed through tax revenues and the uncertainty from year to year of both eligibility and benefits discontinued (Eilers, 1971).

In 1970, the United States spent a great deal less and a much smaller proportion of our gross national product on health care than we do now. There were relatively few Americans enrolled in health maintenance organizations. Most physicians, there were less of them relative to the population, were in solo practice and were paid on a fee-for service basis. Neither hospitals nor physician specialists were in oversupply. Then as now, quality of care was uneven, with access variable, and with service which was not customer focused. Unquestionably there has been a great deal of development of medical technology over the last 28 years since Bob wrote the article, which, although the health status of the American population hasn't improved relative to that of other developed countries, more effective medical care has certainly improved the functioning and even the life expectancies of millions of Americans.

Implementation of the Eilers proposal, or something like it, would have saved the country billions of dollars (which, it is true, wouldn't have been earned by those working in the health care sector). Adoption would have led to greater increases in quality, more even distribution of care, less dissatisfaction with health delivery, and obviously more equitable insurance coverage. Other people's proposals may have had the same effect. And the Eilers proposal would have been fought against too by the organized forces of insurance, hospitals, and medicine.

Eilers' approach was well reasoned, advanced for its time, and sensitive to political nuances. The criteria encouraged competition, with limited regulation by government. Providers were not told what to do and how to do it; rather they were to be guided by the demands and expectations of knowledgeable purchasers and regulators. Better results in delivering health care were rewarded as the more productive and entrepreneurial provider organizations obtained more of the business. Most health policy academics do not favor an Eilers-type approach. This is for a variety of reasons, political and otherwise.

Bob would probably have responded to his critics, "This may not be the best plan, but it is less bad than the other plans. Show me how to improve it, and let's work it through together." What scuttled the Clinton plan for national health insurance, other than its complexity and lack of due process, was the President's unwillingness to take on employers who currently don't provide their employees with adequate health insurance and are unwilling to pay for it. Will paying for such health insurance raise the cost of doing business? Certainly, and so what? At least, those employers providing health benefits to their employees and the uninsured and their families should favor a plan for universal health insurance that is simple and understandable. The acceptable national health plan: (1) insures all Americans; (2) limits what government will pay; (3) encourages competition among effective provider organizations; and (4) is phased in, to get the bugs out of the plan, and to transition those organizations and workers whose services will no longer be required.

What Did We Set Out to Do?

By 1967, an active interest had developed within the School of Medicine and the Wharton School for establishing structural relationships through which faculty members in both divisions of the University of Pennsylvania could join for research activities as well as educational programs. This led to establishment of the Leonard Davis Institute of Health Economics in 1967, which was funded by a New Yorker who had made a fortune as principal owner of Colonial Penn Insurance Company.

One of the initial decisions was that the Institute would not have an independent faculty. Rather, faculty members from existing departments at the University would commit specific amounts of time, whether research or instructional, to its work, which would be paid for by the Institute. In the new Master's program in Health Care Administration, the successful candidate would receive his or her degree from the Wharton School. The Leonard Davis Institute acted in the capacity of an academic department relative to the program in health care administration. (The program later became an academic department, of Health Care Systems.)

In 1967, a decision was made at Penn to establish a Department of Community Medicine in the medical school. Also, at that time, the University of Pennsylvania Medical Center was also formed, composed of seven independent hospitals with 3,000 teaching beds. Courses in the new Wharton program were made available to medical students (although they could not easily enroll because of the bad fit between the medical and business school calendars). Occasional medical school graduates did become able to and participated in joint MD/MBA and MD/PhD programs. In an article written by Bob Eilers, Bill Kissick, chair of Community Medicine, and myself for the Association of University Programs in Health Administration, in May 1970, my selection as program director was announced, as follows:

The collaborative nature of this endeavor is dramatized in the selection of the program Director, Dr. Anthony Kovner. A Ph.D. in (sic) Medical Care Administration from the School of Public and International Affairs of the University of Pittsburgh, he has had several years of management experience in the Beth Israel Hospital and the Gouverneur Health Services program in New York City. Dr. Kovner was recruited to Penn in September, 1969 to assume planning and administrative responsibilities in the Department of Medicine, with a teaching and research base in the Department of Community Medicine . . . His joint faculty appointment in the Wharton School plus continuing management responsibility in the University of Pennsylvania Medical Center indicates the determination to effect close collaboration between management and medicine at Penn. (Kovner, Eilers, & Kissick, 1970)

The academic program conducted over 2 years at Wharton required five core courses in accounting, statistics, administration, economic analysis and policy, and quantitative methods (as was required for all Wharton students). The six health care courses required were: (1) Structure and Organization of the Health Services Enterprise, (2) Health Care Administration, (3) Community Medicine and Health Planning, (4) Health Care Costs, (5) Health Care Financing, and (6) Decision-Making in Health Care Administration. Students could take six electives and had to take a research seminar, and a three-month summer residency between the two academic years. Electives included personnel and labor management, data processing, operations analysis, legal aspects of health care administration, social entrepreneurship, and other Wharton courses. Ideal enrollment was viewed as 35 entering students each year, but of course we started much smaller. (The first "class" had only four students.)

What was new or different about the program at the time? Not much. It was being offered at the prestigious Wharton School, and sponsored as well by the Penn Medical School. Not being a department was a political move to overcome the objections of other departments. I suppose what was most distinctive about the program was its very existence at Wharton, in its own redesigned building shared with the insurance department in the middle of the campus, with our own classrooms and meeting rooms. Significant, too, was that leadership of the program was coming out of the insurance sector. Insurance had not been and is not a key component of competitor health administration programs, many of which are in schools of public health. (At NYU, as of 1998, we did not even have a course in health care financing, although the subject is covered in part in the course in health economics and payment systems.)

An obvious defect of the approach at Penn was that we were constrained to recruit those faculty members in other departments who wanted to join with us (or be bought out) rather than recruiting the best from a national pool. Whomever we did recruit still had to obtain tenure in their own department, and these were primarily junior professors. Only Dr. Kissick remains, as of 1998, in the department of Health Systems, and he is primarily a medical school faculty member. Of the 13 faculty in our original group, six left the university, one retired, two are deceased, and three have remained at Penn but are in other departments in which they obtained tenure and are not part of the Health Systems department. The Penn program is currently one of the finest in the United States and in the world, both in research and in teaching.

What Did I Learn at Penn?

Most of what I learned at Penn is not about health care management. I learned a great deal about how universities are organized and how universities, schools, and departments function. As organizations, universities have a lot in common with hospitals. This is because of their nonprofit sponsorship and because of the relative autonomy of the principal professional workers.

Academic departments within universities work on the basis of tenure (obviously this is not the case for physicians in private practice). Professors are tenured primarily based on their scholarly achievements, which are measured principally by single-authored publications in peer reviewed journals. Merit is reviewed at the department level, at the school level, and at Penn by a committee appointed by the president, and then by the president. Because this is a job for life, hurdles are constructed. At Penn, the two key points in the process are the departmental review and the Presidential Special Committee review. The "best" peer-reviewed journals typically focus on articles in one discipline (such as economics) and are theory-preferential (such as the *Administrative Science Quarterly*).

At Penn in 1970, the work of the health care administration program mostly militated against me, or someone like me getting tenure. I didn't get my Ph.D. in an academic discipline. I had been hired as a manager (and was still working as a manager, part-time, in the medical school), and I had to work to get the program organized and eventually accredited by the Association for Accrediting Graduate Programs in health care administration. Most of my other work was teaching, and I worked as a consultant with Bob Eilers, for his private company.

What Did I Learn at Penn About Teaching Health Care Management?

At Wharton, the main course that I taught (and which I still teach) was called Health Care Administration. I had taken such a course at Cornell, in 1962, with Fred LeRocker, which consisted largely in the anecdotes of a retired hospital administrator reviewing his experiences with the various departments that had been in his hospital—medical, nursing, medical records, housekeeping, engineering, and so forth. Perhaps my memory is faulty regarding how Professor LeRocker's management class was organized. Most certainly he spent considerable time dealing with the relationship of physicians in private practice to the management and board of the nonprofit hospital.

There was no equivalent course, at the time, in the general management specialization at Wharton. The closest approximation was probably a "production" course, as management courses at that time were more concerned with manufacturing than with services. The topics covered in my course were The Health Care (HC) Manager, Education of the HC Manager, Goals, Governance, Interorganizational Structure, Organizational Structure, Medical Staff, Productivity, Nonprofessionals, Patients, and Community. Several weeks of the semester were devoted to team presentations.

One innovation I made was to organize the 35 students into six teams. Each team related to a local health care institution, with whose management I had developed a relationship for the course. Each team was to interview managers at the assigned unit and later make a class presentation on the current level of unit performance, desired performance, what the manager could do to improve unit performance, priorities, and recommendations. Presentations were rehearsed with me prior to the class. In addition, each team member, with the consultation of the group, had to prepare a written report on one of the following topics: goals of the unit, power structure of the units, interorganizational structure, organizational structure, integration of professional staff and unit goals, productivity or efficiency of the unit, and the relation of the unit to those served by the unit. There were no examinations. Grades were on the following basis: class participation 50%, unit report 25% and class presentation 25%, on which the team was graded as a unit.

In reviewing the 1974 readings, there were 33 articles and 6 case studies. At least a third of these articles and cases were written by me or someone I knew well, often about an organization in which I had worked. Several of the selected articles had made a great impression on me as a doctoral student (and I think still make good reading today). These included Cyert and March's (1964) piece on organizational goals, Perrow's (1963) case study on goals and power structure, Gordon's (1961) article on "Top Management Triangle in Voluntary Hospitals," Starkweather's (1970) piece on the "Rationalization for Decentralization in Large Hospitals", Mechanic's (1962) "Sources of Power of Lower Participants in Complex Organizations," and Strauss's (1972) "Hospital Organization from the Viewpoint of Patient Centered Goals."

As an example of how I was influenced by these articles, I will examine more closely an aspect of Cyert and March's work. In treating "organizational goals," they viewed the organization as a coalition of individuals who have substantially different preference orderings (individual goals). Coalition members bargain with each other to form goals, with side payments or policy commitments representing the central process of goal specification. Attention to goals is limited, which explains the absence of any strong pressure to resolve apparent internal inconsistencies. "Organizational slack" (excess of organizational resources to payments to the coalition) stabilizes the system during good times by absorbing excess resources and retarding upward adjustment of aspirations, and during bad times slack permits aspirations to be maintained by providing a pool of emergency resources. Goals are therefore a series of more or less independent constraints imposed on the organization through a process of bargaining among potential coalition members and elaborated over time in response to short run pressures.

In the case of health care administration, it is the ruling coalition of a hospital, then, rather than "the hospital" which has goals. There can be a lot of unresolved conflict among goals, such as research, teaching, service, and community benefit. Another example is the presence of "side payments" which explain the existence of "special" projects. Implications for the health care manager include paying attention to the preferences of the ruling coalition and focusing effort on accomplishing their objectives and the difficulties of goal attainment or efforts which lie outside the coalition's attention. Theory explained, therefore, through focus and logic much of the muddle of managerial politics I had previously been involved with at Beth Israel and Gouverneur and which I was observing now at the University of Pennsylvania Medical Center.

A hallmark of my teaching then (and now) was to view management as an art or craft rather than as a science. I emphasized three aspects of the learning process: (1) interaction between class participants and the teacher, (2) the inclusion of experience with the real world of health care organizations, and (3) development of oral and written presentation skills. At that time at the Wharton School, this was not being done in most other classes (in any classes, so far as I remember) or in most other programs of health care administration.

Teaching is one of the hardest things to do well and is one of the easiest things to do poorly. To teach well, one must have a command of the subject, be a wonderful performer, and be sensitive to the particular skills and experience of a particular class. Bob Eilers gave me a number of useful pointers: the importance of knowing everyone's name, coming to class with a few well-chosen questions to ask the students, and inviting all the students over at the end of the semester for a formal dinner.

What Did I Learn at Penn About Doing Research?

One of the best strategies for an academic, as Bob Eilers advised me, is to choose a delimited field and become an expert. I chose the topic of nonprofit boards and how they contribute to hospital performance. This topic was useful to me because not much scholarly research had been published, and because of the practical benefits if I ever became a CEO working with a nonprofit board.

Because my Ph.D. was in an applied field rather than in a discipline— I had never intended to become an academic—I knew that achieving tenure would be particularly difficult in my case. From the onset, Bob Eilers told me that if I were to get tenure I would have to produce quality research published in the best journals. He did not tell me the quantity of articles that was expected—not that there was any specific number. Bob told me that he would look after me and help me as much as he could, which satisfied me.

I chose to examine the role of hospital boards in making policy. I surveyed board members of 47 large hospitals in southeastern Pennsylvania and southwestern New Jersey concerning their assessments of: (1) board power relative to the executive director, (2) key hospital priority areas for the next three years, and (3) their qualifications to make decisions in these priority areas. I made three major findings: First, relative to other operational areas, a greater number of governing board members assigned high priority to cost control, quality control, and relations with third-party payers. Second, perceived qualifications to make decisions in all operational areas varied with the occupations of the board members. And third, a greater proportion of physicians and administrators as compared with other occupational groups rated themselves as very well qualified in operational areas relating to medical care programs and in relations with special agencies affecting hospital reimbursement and expansion.

My main advice to doctoral students is to choose and gain access to good data which has not been previously analyzed. The first difficulty, of course, is getting good data. Getting such data is a twofold process that requires gaining access to the organization, and getting the data from those who can give it to you. This has been especially difficult in my case, because hospital trustees do not participate without the agreement of their CEO, to whom the benefits of such a study often seem dubious at best. Indeed, if a study comes up with any real findings, such findings would most likely be negative concerning the performance or qualifications of trustees. Therefore, such research is not generally seen as worthwhile of support.

My research was published in *Medical Care*, one of the best journals in the field, and I made the following observations in my discussion of the findings. The literature at that time was saying that hospital boards were supposed to make hospital policy, which was carried out by administrators. To perform this role, I suggested that board members should be qualified by virtue of expertise and experience and have available time and necessary information. According to my data, the board members surveyed said that they *did* make major policy decisions and that they *were* qualified to make major decisions. They said they felt very well qualified to make policy decisions in areas relating to financial performance and community and labor relations as compared with areas relating to medical care programs and special agencies which influenced hospital reimbursement and expansion.

I concluded that assuming that governing boards do make major policy decisions and should continue doing so, and that operational areas for hospitals relating to medical care programs and special agencies would become increasingly important, that boards should select new members with expertise in the key priority areas—namely, physicians and administrators. I suggested that the gap between board priorities and qualifications of trustees indicated that board composition should be changed periodically, that a committee of the governing board be charged with the self-evaluation function, and that the addition of new members with required expertise in operational areas would be facilitated by limiting terms of office for all board members.

I was pleased to have carried out a major research study; after all, I had done a great deal of work, and the article, after having been reviewed by peers, was found suitable for publication in a respected academic journal. If my findings were not revolutionary, or national, trustees said what I believed they were going to say, which had practical implications. On the other hand, I hoped that trustees hadn't checked off "well qualified" for each of ten questions when there were four options also including "very well qualified," "poorly qualified," and "very poorly qualified." I also wondered whether "quality control," (e.g., programs to reduce medication errors) was a topic that the board should be making policy in. Could the board be expected to know a great deal about quality control? What did they understand "quality control" to mean?

Why Did I Leave Penn?

I left because I did not receive tenure. The committee had found my publications record unsatisfactory and there was nothing Bob Eilers could do. Disappointed and surprised, with a new wife, a one-year-old, and a baby on the way, I felt I had to leave Penn quickly. I was 38 years old. What had I learned from my experience at Penn? Now, I believe, not enough. At Penn, I had learned how to start and run a graduate program in health care administration. I also thought that I didn't want to be an academic. I knew I didn't want to be an assistant hospital administrator. What was I to do?

Reflection: On Teaching and Research in Management

To what extent are and should managers be teachers? What is the connection between program evaluation or planning and management research? Drucker (1999) indicates that some people learn best by writing, others by reading, some by listening, others by talking. Do academics learn best by writing and reading, while managers learn best by listening and by talking? Consider the following examples of different kinds of managers. Are they more effective to the extent that they are better teachers and researchers?

1. Henry Lopez sees himself as a "servant manager" providing advice and counsel to frontline doctors and nurses in their work of treating patients. He spends a great deal of time talking with doctors and nurses and with patients and potential patients to find out their perceptions of service and their attitudes toward the organization.

2. Bill Brown manages accounts receivables and is trying to figure out what are the best measures for effectiveness in his work. He also seeks to

know with what other organizations should he be comparing his results to, and how he can best get the workers in his department to take more "ownership" of their jobs rather than merely carrying out his instructions.

3. Lana Borukhova, manager of ambulatory care, is trying to develop a management education program for the physicians who practice in her very large, urban program. She wants to find out what they need to know, who best can teach them, and how to pay for the program. Most of the physicians with whom she works have very little understanding of managed care, or even of basic supervisory techniques, and yet they are expected to manage risk and function in teams.

Many managers do not see being an effective teacher as part of their job description. But obviously if managers are going to work with others rather than do all the work themselves, they have to be able to get those who work with them to learn. Teaching is related to being able to reflect upon the work that managers do, and then testing what you have learned with those with whom you work or with those who understand your work.

As a functional specialist, the manager must master some discipline or body of techniques, such as statistics, operations research, finance, or marketing. I don't believe that all health care managers have to know all these techniques equally well. But all need to know the language in these areas and be able to ask good questions about the validity and reliability of assumptions and techniques.

Working in a nonprofit academic institution has similarities to working in a nonprofit health care institution, and obviously some nonprofit health care organizations also have educational and research missions. Working in an academic health center is obviously different from working in a community organization with no main mission of education and research. Academic health centers are much more complex because of the salience of the different missions whose proponents vie for scarce resources and mission protection. I believe in at least budgetary separation of the three missions of service, teaching, and research, for accountability and protection purposes. When this isn't done in academic health centers the result is often tangled bureaucracy and paralysis in the face of hostile environments.

What academic health centers have going for them, besides a lot of smart, dedicated people, is the importance of mission and the richness of experience for young managers trying to figure out what they're really good at, and what they really want to do. For obvious reasons, they are usually less profit-driven than some health care organizations and less service-driven than others.

What teaching management and doing research about management has in its favor, as a career, especially in an academic environment, is more control of your time (after seven or eight years of heavy apprenticeship post PhD). There is less financial reward, and, obviously, greater opportunities to teach and do research about management if that is what you like doing. Unfortunately too little research and teaching in health care management is produced jointly by practitioners and academics, and quality suffers thereby, not only in the university, but also in practice. The effective manager is always teaching those whom he works with, those whom he or she sells to and buys from. The effective manager uses disciplined research approaches to get the data he/she needs, to evaluate data, to make management decisions based on specified assumptions, comparing action alternatives based on financial and other constraints, and learning stakeholder preferences and expectations.

Learning About Teaching and Research in Health Services Management

Yes	No	
___	___	Do you think that it is important for health care managers to be good teachers?
___	___	Do you have a good idea of your effectiveness as a teacher?
___	___	Do you seek opportunities to teach and gain feedback as to your teaching skills?
___	___	Do you regularly read journals which take a scientific approach to aspects of health services management?
___	___	Do you have regular discussions with experts regarding what data you need in your job and how to get it?
___	___	Do you regularly take advantage of continuing education opportunities in some aspect of health services management?
___	___	Do you know and respect several health services managers who are effective teachers and researchers?

Practical Exercise

First, develop a learning contract for the next 12 months that involves practicing your teaching skills and getting feedback as to your skills attainment. (For example, volunteer to teach part of your organization's orientation program.) Second, write an article for publication in a selected health services journal. Review the literature about the topic you wish to write about and share an outline of the proposed paper with one of your former teachers or colleagues. Then collect and analyze data about the unit in which you are working. Share your work with colleagues and mentors. One such project might deal with performance indicators for your unit. What are they now? What problems or concerns do you have with these indicators? What recommendations would you make for different indicators? If implemented, what impact do the new indicators have on unit performance?

5

Laboring for the Union

The older I got, and the more experience I had, the harder it was to find a suitable job. Somebody told me once that it took a month for each $10,000 in salary to find a suitable job. In 1974, I became senior health consultant for the United Autoworkers. I found the job through a colleague of my brother Joel's. (Joel was employed by the Kaiser-Permanente Health Plan in Los Angeles.) He worked with Avram Yedidia, an elderly and influential consultant, who worked for Kaiser. Avram's friend Mel Glasser, director of the Social Security Department for the United Autoworkers, was looking to fill a replacement position, preferably someone with an advanced degree, who knew something about health care, and who was willing to learn the "union" part.

What was there that appealed to me about this job? There was nothing in my background that was pro-union. My father was a manager and an owner, and I identified with my father and his interests. I liked the idea of working for what I saw as a consumer organization, fighting the good fight for Americans who were buying health insurance and using medical care. I didn't like the idea of living in Detroit where I didn't know anybody, but it was a city not so far away (one hour by plane) from New York. The UAW was looking for somebody with my credentials. I could regard the job as a promotion. It didn't lead anywhere, but I wasn't going anywhere. I could stay at the union, or as before, seek another academic position, or move on into hospital administration, still my preference.

The job requirements were as follows. First, I would have to learn about what the benefits coverage was at the several companies to which I was assigned, the major company being the Ford Motor Company (the UAW also represented workers in the aircraft and the agricultural industries, and in other industries as well, particularly companies who supplied the automobile manufacturers). The benefits coverages for which I was specifically responsible were health and group life insurance. Second, I was to be a leader of the team to evaluate and approve health maintenance organizations (HMOs) which UAW members could join. Third, I was to be involved with Mel Glasser in writing testimony on health legislation for UAW officers. Fourth, I was involved in administrative issues relating to benefits recently negotiated, such as dental, and in the development of new benefit specifications, such as for vision care. Of course, I didn't know anything about any of this at the time. But what Mel Glasser appeared to want was somebody who knew something about health care, someone who was intelligent and could write (and write quickly), someone who could take orders, and be a good teamworker.

Detroit, Michigan

We bought a big house in Grosse Pointe, a suburb of Detroit. Detroit is built, understandably enough, for automobiles. The move was difficult for my family. My wife followed me to Detroit, after delivering our younger daughter Anna, in New York. My first memory of Detroit was a terrific ice storm. It was bitter cold, the sky was gray, and my wife, our two small children, and I had to move in with another family, as our electricity was out for several days. We didn't know anyone in Detroit, except for Chris's former boyfriend's parents, who lived on the other side of town. Most of our neighbors didn't have kids. The only person we knew in our neighborhood was Mel Glasser.

I remember that Detroiters considered themselves Easterners (the same time zone), and that no one appreciated my sense of humor (irony was lost there). Power was concentrated in the business world in a way utterly different from New York. The city of Detroit was going downhill, and parts of Detroit reminded me of the slums in north Philadelphia. Detroiters took themselves very seriously, and they took work very seriously. You had to drive to get anywhere. There was nothing wrong with Detroit, but it wasn't home.

The UAW Social Security Department

Circa 1975, the UAW represented a total of 4.5 million people, including 1.4 million active employees, about 300,000 retirees, and their families, nearly one-third of whom lived in Michigan. The UAW had national collective bargaining contracts with 17 employers, and 3,100 local collective bargaining agreements. The UAW was organized both by national departments (relating to a specific company or set of companies) and by geographic region. There were national departments for Ford, General Motors, Chrysler, and so forth, and 18 regional offices, six of which were in Michigan. The UAW's governing body was a 26-person executive board, with one director from each of the 18 regions, including Canada, and nine international officers. There were about 1,600 local unions in the UAW, ranging in size from a few members to over 30,000 members.

The UAW had a long history of concern with community and public affairs in addition to its interest in workers' pay and benefits. For example, UAW leaders expended a tremendous amount of time and energy advocating national health insurance even though the majority of UAW members already had comprehensive health care benefits. The UAW also had departments for women, retired workers, community relations, and education, among others.

UAW contracts generally provided for service benefits rather than indemnity coverages. After benefits were negotiated, the employer was generally responsible for administration of the benefits program. Insurance carriers, usually Blue Cross and Blue Shield, were generally under contract with the employer to deliver the benefits.

The UAW specified at least five ways of thinking about health benefits and health policy. (1) The UAW supported consumer participation in policy making, first-dollar benefits coverage and uniform implementation of benefits. (2) The Union believed in community rather than union-operated facilities. (3) The UAW was involved in benefits design. (4) The Union was philosophically opposed to for-profit organizations in health care. (5) The UAW believed in comprehensive health care coverage. Standard benefits included 365 days of doctor and hospital inpatient care; 45 days of psychiatric doctor and hospital care; emergency care, outpatient psychiatric care up to $1,000 per year, prescription drugs with a $3 copayment; home care; substance abuse treatment in hospital, in residential facilities (up to 45 days), and up to 35 outpatient visits per year (up to a lifetime maximum of 140 visits); prenatal and postnatal care and pap smears, prosthetic appliances and durable medical equipment and a comprehensive dental care program with 100% plan payments for exams, prophylaxis, and emergencies; 90% for x-rays, extraction and periodontal repairs, restoration and endodontics; and 50% for bridges and dentures up to $750 per person per year, and 50% for orthodontia with a lifetime maximum of $650.

Cost control was important to the UAW, because the money that paid for health care premiums could be directed otherwise to wages or other benefits. The Union favored consumer-controlled prepaid group practice plans. The UAW supported plans whose revenues derived principally from capitation payments and which had adequate quality controls. The UAW opposed for-profit HMOs whose practice consisted of fee-for-service patients side-by-side with capitation patients. The UAW also opposed offering optional choice for HMOs which lacked adequate quality control and consumer participation.

My unit, the Social Security Department, was expected to support the line union departments in collective bargaining and to help shape and rationalize the union's policies on health care and on pensions. We had a staff of about 15 professionals, and were responsible for group life insurance and supplementary job insurance as well as health care and pensions. The senior staff included the aforementioned Mel Glasser, director, whose background was in social work, John Sparks, the deputy director, who was a Canadian and a health expert, Claude Poulin, a French-speaking Canadian, who was the pensions expert, and Manny Bittkau, an experienced negotiator, whose background was mostly on the pensions, and unemployment benefits. In health care, Mel, John, and I were joined by Pat Killeen, a junior associate, who had a master's degree in health care.

Lessons Learned in the Social Security Department

With all of my previous jobs, rather than working my way up through an organization, I had to learn an entire job about which I knew virtually nothing, under the gun. At Gouverneur, I had been flung into battle, as neither my predecessor nor the chief executive were there when I started. At Penn, I was told what to do and had pretty much free rein at Wharton in deciding how it was done. At the UAW, however, the job I filled had been vacant for some time, so there was time to learn on the job.

Assigned to Ford, I spent many hours reading the benefits book—the health care section ran 200 pages alone—and I was supposed to learn group life as well. Pat Killeen knew more about benefits than I did, and I was fortunate that John Sparks and Pat were very patient with me, answering all my questions graciously, despite my repetitions. The UAW Social Security Department was a unit in which I did as I was told, rather than my being empowered to take ownership of my work. This suited my purposes in part, as I was under personal stress—moving to Detroit with young children, and knowing no one. Also because I knew so little about so much of the basics of union business, I traveled less than the more experienced consultants who dealt with the smaller companies.

I spent a great deal of time at Michigan Blue Cross and Blue Shield, the main health care carrier for the "Big Three" auto companies, and some time at the Metropolitan Health Plan (which later merged with Henry Ford Health Plan) as a board member. And I spent time writing first drafts of speeches given by union executives or reviewing policy statements in health care written by others. For the most part, I kept quiet, and listened, a policy I would advise for newcomers in any field. The line union representatives had little to do with me, as they were experts on the implementation of the contracts. Our department was involved in the development and negotiation of benefits, and in approving HMOs for dual choice, in which I soon became heavily involved, both for medical and dental HMOs.

At the UAW, I learned about how a large union works. I learned about how health insurance works and the details of health benefit programs negotiated by employers and unions. I learned how to write a good speech for a union official testifying before congress. I learned how insurance carriers work and about the perspectives of the benefits staff in large corporations. I further developed my own views on health policy. I agreed with the UAW concerning the necessity for national health insurance (although I preferred other plans to the UAW's Health Security bill), consumer participation in policy making, community-operated rather than union-operated facilities, involvement of the union in benefits design, and cost control. Where I disagreed concerned opposition to for-profit organizations in health care, support for first-dollar benefits coverage, and favoring a more principal role for government, particularly of national government in health care.

Negative Response to My Boss

When I knew him 20 years ago, Mel Glasser was about 60 years old, smallish, with coal-black hair and a short black mustache. He reminded me of a Russian bureaucrat of the Anastas Mikoyan variety. He often wore sporty clothes, and was expressive in his facial gestures. Mel was married to a lovely woman and they had children. He was very intelligent and a person of strong convictions. I soon came to dislike him very much, even though I respected his talent and experience.

We differed on a number of issues. Mel saw the for-profits in health care as primarily interested in making money rather than in improving people's health. Numerous scandals had proven that "you cannot trust" the for-profits in health care, which is the people's right, rather than a privilege. Copayments, coinsurance, and deductibles discourage access to medical care for poor people, while they don't affect use by those with higher incomes. Thus, patient direct payment is discriminatory against poor people who should have the same access to medical care as all Americans. State health policy is controlled either by for-profit business corporations that do not have an interest in equal access to health care, or by provider interests that are seeking economic subsidies and protection, often at the expense of the taxpayer, if not the consumer.

Then, there was the memory of Bob Eilers, who had been a model boss (and who had convictions often opposite Mel's, regarding for-profits, first-dollar coverage, and the role of big government). Mel corrected me and everyone else continually in front of others. He also gave me little freedom in my work, and when I had completed it, treated it as his own.

Following are two examples of how it was difficult for me to work for him. I always had to keep my door open, so that he could see to whom I was talking. And he read everybody's mail before we received it (my wife suggested sending me a love letter from someone else and see what Mel would do with it.) Also, I saw him lie repeatedly, to promote what he defined as UAW interests, in conversations with third parties, most particularly with the auto companies, for example, regarding what the evidence was on the effect of coinsurance and deductibles on access to care. I also objected to his taking credit for my work, written for union officials, and giving it to them as if it was his own work.

The current dean of NYU's Wagner School, Jo Boufford, in a lecture recently, said that a manager should always have an exit strategy from a job and know what the line is over which she/he will refuse to do something. If she/he cannot be loyal to her/his boss, she/he should quit the job. This strategy can be difficult to implement in practice. In my case, I had just accepted this UAW job and moved to Detroit, and I had a wife and young children to support. I was also learning, and this was a good job. Mel traveled often and so did I (at least I was out of the building) and the union line people with whom I worked didn't like Mel either, nor did many of the staff in his own department. John Sparks, however, worshipped Mel (Pat liked him too), because Mel knew what was right, was able, and had fought the good fight, while the people he was fighting against would stop at nothing to harm the workers. I was extremely fond of John Sparks, who was the most knowledgeable person I had ever met concerning health benefits, particularly those he had designed, such as the dental plan. John was totally honest, never criticized anyone publicly, and was always helpful and supportive. He never took credit for someone else's work. Perhaps this is somehow why the two of them got along so well. Mel criticized John, never gave him credit, but John didn't seem to notice. John had a wonderful sense of humor. Mel liked a good laugh too. Many of Mel's views were so out of sync with the American body politic, which Mel never acknowledged. He assumed that union leaders knew what was best for union members, and that Mel, as the expert, knew what was best regarding health benefits and plans. Mel so informed the union leaders who then informed the rank and file.

My Views on the Issues

Mel and I agreed substantively on a wide range of issues, such as the desirability (although we accorded it different priority) of getting accurate information from the companies on the cost, use, and quality of the health benefits program. At that time, the companies' data was almost wholly limited to what the program cost them, and information was compiled relative to contracts of individual workers rather than to those who were covered, which included the workers' family members.

Some UAW members got even better coverage than that stipulated under the contracts, as the insurance carrier routinely approved denied coverage when pressured to do so by line union officials who were not above threatening to replace the insurer, if they didn't approve coverage.

I agreed with Mel that there had been major scandals involving the for-profits in health care, but also there had been major scandals involving nonprofits. The major variance among provider or carrier performance does not flow from sponsorship. There are excellent for-profits and lousy nonprofits. Why not judge every organization based on its performance, not its sponsorship? Focus attention on the way performance is measured, and generate information specific enough to judge performance.

With regard to copays, I agreed with Mel that copays affected use, but often this was in the direction of discouraging wasteful use rather than preventing persons from getting needed care. In any event, all Americans were not entitled to the same free health care coverage, anymore than they were entitled to the same free education coverage. Although everyone is entitled to grade school, not everyone is entitled to a PhD. So, it made sense to me to have copays for certain health services and up to certain amounts, to discourage wasteful use. Taxpayers or premium payers can't afford to provide all the health benefits all Americans want, and obviously the current system skews billions into health care that might have been better spent on education, infrastructure, or on higher wages.

In the United States, health care is largely the responsibility of the states. (Medicare is an exception.) The United States is a very large country, with a dispersed population, and the people in Idaho may want and should have and are willing to pay for a very different health care system than the citizens of New York City. I believe and have argued in favor of fixed budgets for capitated health care rather than paying for health care only in a fee-for-service way. This is because capitation forces providers and consumers to determine priorities in spending limited resources. I do believe that drugs, mental health, and chronic care should be inside the circle and paid for under the capitation rate, but certainly not all drugs, not all mental health services, and not all chronic care.

Lessons Learned About Management at the UAW

I learned little about management at the UAW. I learned that different management styles could be equally effective, by witnessing Mel Glasser's style, which differed greatly from Bob Eilers'. Yet he was equally effective. I learned something of the importance of the internal politics of unions to the collective bargaining process. A union officer who is fighting to retain his elected job, or another union officer trying to get control of a region, affects negotiations between companies and unions. The UAW had difficulties of its own in negotiating with a different clerical union that had organized employees working at headquarters prior to my working there. So unions themselves are employers, facing the same management challenges as do other organizations. The UAW had been and was losing members nationally and losing political clout because it was losing members. Why this was so was related to national trends—as the percentage of American workers in unions was decreasing, most particularly in the private sector. The auto companies would argue that the UAW had negotiated such high wages and benefits that this made the companies less competitive resulting in job losses, and this prevented unions from organizing workers in other industries.

On this last point, I have come to the conclusion that workers should mainly be paid based on profit sharing, whether unionized or not. This lowers wage costs in difficult times and gives workers a stake in the increasing profits that accompany good times. (I believe in profit sharing for nonprofit and governmental organizations as well.) And I believe in full sharing of information regarding what all workers are paid, and how each unit of an organization contributes to the organization's financial success or lack of same.

My stance on unions is similar to that taken earlier for profit organizations in health care. There are some unions which are good for the worker and the employer and some which are not. Many organizations have benefitted from being unionized, as their workers were being exploited. As a manager, I would rather not deal with a union because this is an added cost of production and because this adds an extra level of difficulty to the decision-making process. But I would prefer having a union than to fighting a union during an organizing process and still having to get out the work at the same time. To the extent that an organization has difficulties in managing and succeeding in the market and blames this on unions, my usual response would be to blame management. Management has an equal say in the bargaining process and in the implementation of the contract, unless of course management is at a tremendous disadvantage in bargaining because of the industry power of a large union.

Reflection: Working with Unions

To what extent do unions help and hinder managers? To what extent do unions exploit and protect union members? Can the manager learn from experience in working with unions to deal more effectively with other stakeholder groups, such as community advocates, physicians, board members, nurses, and with other managers? Here are some examples of the kinds of situations that working with a union can illuminate:

1. Noel Knowles, a city hospital administrator, tells Brian Kent, a health care administration student, "Don't work in a city hospital if you have any other alternative open to you. You just can't get anything done because of the unions. The union got my last boss fired because he was trying to get the right things done."
2. Bill Appleton, a union official, is insisting that the hospital with whom the union contracts guarantee the jobs of the union's members, and allocate sufficient monies to retrain union members, as needed, to meet the changing demands for health care.
3. Sheila Kent, a salaried internist in ambulatory care at an urban medical center, is unhappy with the hospital bureaucracy and how her requests for improved service and outreach have largely been neglected. She is thinking of joining a union.

What reasons are there for a union if an organization is well-managed? Perhaps none, but perhaps also most health care organizations aren't managed well enough. Does the union function then to get the workers the best salaries and benefits and to give employees the best job protection? Do unions necessarily hate managers? Or do they merely see managers as being on the other side, much as rival basketball players do, or lawyers who function as plaintiffs and defense attorneys, competing on the court or in court and then able to eat together afterwards companionably.

The question for most managers is how to work most effectively with the unions in the workplace, rather than how they can work most effectively to keep unions out that they don't want. Assuming that there is a union, it makes sense for the manager to treat the union's representatives just as he/she would treat any other organized group. As with community advocates, the manager should attempt to get to know the union representatives better. This includes understanding the existing labor agreement (about which the union people are likely to be experts), knowing what are "hot" issues for the leadership and for the membership, understanding something about union politics (Are there issues in union elections being contested by whom on what basis?).

Managers need to understand their own feelings about working with union workers and leaders. Are these people whom the manager doesn't believe to be reasonable, i.e. "The union isn't fair and doesn't try to be fair to management." Managers should know what union leaders can and cannot do now and over time in providing better and more efficient service to patients. Can the manager fire a union worker whom he observes is rude to a patient? How can the manager reward individual union members who are doing a fine job?

How can management work with a unionized labor force to improve productivity, quality, and service? Is this feasible with more or less the same or with a reduced labor force? I know there are companies that have improved performance a great deal working together with union leaders. Sensenbrenner observed during his mayoral experience in Madison, Wisconsin, that "some wary union leaders and members turned out to be among my strongest backers." The union president told Sensenbrenner that "Before the quality program, all we did was put out fires . . . The message from management was . . . do as you're told." Once the program was well underway, however, the message became, "You and your teammates understand your work better than management can. Tell us how to help you do it better." (Sensenbrenner, 1991)

There are no easy answers to preparing unions and managers to work with each other as colleagues and partners. What is important is to deal with issues with open minds. In my experience, most problems with unions are also problems with management. No one expects management and unions to agree about everything or about most things, but it is reasonable to expect them to agree that most organizations must respond to what the market demands in order to survive and flourish, and that workers and managers have a mutual interest in working together to see that the organization survives and flourishes.

Reflection: Learning About Working with Unions

Yes	No	
_____	_____	Do you think unions are "never any good?"
_____	_____	Do you think unions are a main reason why unionized health care organizations perform less well than they should?
_____	_____	Do you know enough about what your union does for its members and about how union officers are elected on what platforms?
_____	_____	Can you identify what are the main problems and concerns with your existing labor contracts?
_____	_____	Are you familiar with the discussions which surrounded your organization's last union contractual agreements?
_____	_____	Are you familiar with the views of the workforce who are most pro-union?
_____	_____	Are you sufficiently familiar with the views of non-unionized workers who would be most likely to vote for a union?

Practical Exercise

Read carefully the contract provisions for job security in one of your union contracts. Do you think that the union workers could attain their current degree of job security without union representation? Consider some stakeholder group in your organization, such as physicians or nurses, which currently is not unionized. What expectations do they have of the organization and how well are their expectations being met? In what ways does management act accountably toward these stakeholder groups and how well do managers communicate with leaders of these groups? Would nonrepresented clinicians be better served by a union? Why or why not?

6

Hospital Chief Executive, But Not for Long

In 1977, Anytown was a city of 55,000 people in a rural area. Its main industries were farming, clothing manufacturing, and trucking. Downtown shopping had been replaced by a shopping mall. The population was about 25% Italian, 25% Hispanic, and 50% all else, mostly middle and low-middle income. For me, Anytown was a strange place to live and work, as I had been brought up in a large city. What soon struck me about the place was that so many people, although presumably friendly, were so concerned to keep others out of their church, their club, or their neighborhood.

Anytown Hospital

Anytown Hospital had about 200 beds, which made it larger than each of the hospitals in the two neighboring smaller towns. The three towns were separate communities, which in important ways viewed each others as rivals for health care resources rather than as allies to improve the health of the greater community. The hospital building took up a large square block. On the other sides of the streets were physician offices. The hospital had basic, secondary medical and surgical services. Many of the voluntary attending medical staff had attended foreign medical schools, and most seemed to be doing well enough financially. Most of the physical facilities were up to date, and the hospital was in fairly good financial shape. Medical care was of variable quality as was nursing care. Most of the nurses had been educated locally in community colleges and hospital nursing schools.

Why and How Did I Get There?

Less than pleased with the Midwest and working for the union, I sought a position as a hospital administrator, a position that I had always wanted to hold. A friend recommended me for the position at Anytown, and I was accepted. Once they offered me the position, discussion ensued concerning salary and benefits. We disagreed about salary—I sought what comparable managers made—and they wanted the title of the position to be executive director (and CEO) rather than president, which was fine with me.

I was somewhat worried about the size of the town, but I thought it would be a good first job as a hospital administrator, and I hoped soon to get a CEO job at a bigger place in a more desirable location. The chair of the board was a respected business executive working in a nearby large city, and the chief of the Medical Staff was a respected physician who had aspirations for the hospital being the best—which was my aspiration as well.

Organizational and Management Structure

Anytown was a nonprofit, short-term, general hospital. The board of trustees had about 20 members—mostly white, male, businessmen, bankers, and lawyers ages 55–70, who knew relatively little about the hospital business. Approximately 100 physicians served on the medical staff. The medical staff used the hospital differentially, as in all hospitals, depending upon their medical specialty. For example, surgery was hospital-based; dermatology was not. Physicians in four medical specialties were "geographic full-time" medical support specialties—anesthesiology, radiology, pathology, and emergency services. Physicians practicing in these specialties were not really in the independent practice of medicine, as opposed to surgeons, internists, cardiologists, and others who saw patients in their private offices. The hospital usually billed for these four services, and in return, the physicians received payment by the hospital in different ways—separate fee-for service billing in anesthesiology, percentage of gross for radiologists, and salary for pathology and emergency medicine.

Over 500 employees worked at Anytown, including technicians and support service staff, in a few large and many small departments. Nursing, finance and billing, housekeeping, and dietary comprised the larger departments. Nursing made up 25% of the hospital budget—over 200 nurses worked at Anytown in about ten nursing units. Smaller departments included biomedical engineering, public relations and development, volunteers, and pastoral. The employees were not unionized.

The hospital was organized as a "professional bureaucracy," with most of the work being done by physicians and nurses and support staff, with relatively little emphasis on technostructure (developing and implementing standards) and middle management. Thus, Anytown was characterized by the typical weaknesses of professional bureaucracies: inability to deal with incompetent and unconscientious professionals; not being well-suited to innovation; and, resistance of physicians to direct supervision and mutual adjustment as infringements on professional autonomy.

My Circumstances As Anytown CEO

Not surprisingly, the kinds of problems I was at first confronted with were financial. Before taking the job, I sought the advice of two experts in the field—one a top executive in a large for-profit firm and the other a professor of management in the Midwest. The top executive advised me always to raise prices as high as possible. He believed that this was the key to running a successful hospital business, especially if patients had pretty much no where else to go and Anytown was their community hospital. The professor told me to be wary of quality problems with the medical staff, as this could get the hospital into trouble. He believed that it was especially important for the medical staff to review charts of new physicians seeking admitting and operating privileges.

There were five major problems: (1) costs being over the state budget ceilings, (2) unfair contracts (for the hospital) with the radiologists, (3) and (4) ineffective department heads and staff vacancies, and (5) the uneven quality of medical care. Anytown was in a highly regulated state, and expenses were over the permitted reimbursement limits with regard to many of the categories of expenditures, e.g. a hospital of a certain size and patient acuity could spend just so much on nursing salaries. The radiologists' contract was up for renewal. I felt that it was ridiculous to continue to pay radiologists a percentage of the gross (there was no incentive for collections and many patients did not pay); whereas the radiologists argued that they had no confidence in the hospital finance department to collect everything that was coming to them, nor in management regarding cost allocation for radiology billing. Then there was the problem of getting state approval and financing for a CT scanner and obtaining new equipment. A particular problem with radiology was the chief of service, a highly volatile, some would say paranoid, individual.

Other problematic individuals were the heads of personnel and public relations. The chief of the Medical Staff pressed to get rid of the director of nursing whom he felt was too business oriented and not sufficiently educated or interested in improving the quality of nursing. We had two vacancies: chief financial officer and chief of emergency services, and we were considering recruiting a neurosurgeon and a neurologist.

I was informed, primarily by the physicians, of the following problems in the quality of medical care: some of the surgeons were "butchers," the obstetrics-gynecology group "cared only about patient revenues and not about patients," several of the general practitioners were "not qualified," for example, referring all patients to specialists (even though these GPs billed for care) because they didn't know how to take care of routine ailments for which patients were or were not appropriately hospitalized. I was told about two older physicians in particular who were older and had reduced their practices. One of whom was said to fall asleep in the operating room, the second to lack knowledge of modern medicine. A third physician was commonly on-call while fishing over 50 miles away from the hospital. One more problematic individual was on staff—a physician who murdered his wife and buried her in his backyard.

Positive circumstances also existed. I liked the two persons largely responsible for hiring me, the chair of the board and the president of the Medical Staff, dedicated, intelligent and experienced individuals, who had chosen me; and, there were no serious financial difficulties or malpractice suits or local hospital competitors.

A Case Study in Hospital Governance

I have told this story elsewhere in a case study called "Whose Hospital," in which a group of doctors and nurses deliver a petition to the board demanding CEO Don Wherry's resignation because he was "incompetent, devious, lacked leadership, had shown unprofessional conduct, and had committed negligent acts." In the case study, I lay out the story in Wherry's rebuttal statement:

> First, I'd like to go through the state of the hospital, as it was when I got here.... There was bad leadership in the nursing department and in several other departments, a lack of medical staff leadership, and few competent department heads ... I have been busy with the finances of the hospital and in improving external relationships with the Hispanics, state officials, and other groups.... Next, it's quite unusual for someone to have to defend

himself on the spot to a list of specific charges which I have been waiting for these past 13 days and just have been made aware of now. I think the way this whole thing has been handled by the doctor and nurse ringleaders is disgraceful. The charges they have made are largely not true and could not be proven even if they were true. Even if the charges are true to a substantial extent, there is still not sufficient reason for your discharging me, certainly not suddenly as they are demanding you to.

The doctors are out to get me because I'm doing the job you've been paying me to do, what I'm evaluated on, and for which I received a very good evaluation and a big raise at the end of last year, presumably because I was doing a good job. Certainly none of you have told me to stop doing what I have been doing to assure quality, contain costs, and improve service. During the past year I gathered information for the medical staff on a new reappointment worksheet so that reappointments aren't made on a rubber stamp process every two years. I pointed out the problems that the low inpatient census in pediatrics would create in retaining beds in the years to come. I obtained model rules and regulations for the medical staff and shared these with the president. I questioned the effectiveness of the tissue committee, which hasn't been meeting, and when it has met, whose minutes are perfunctory. I questioned the performance of the audit committee after our delegated status was placed in question by a visiting physician. I suggested we explore mandated physician donations to the hospital, as was passed and implemented two years ago by a neighboring hospital. When patients made complaints about doctors I took these up with the respective chiefs of departments. I investigated the assertion by a lab technician that tests were being reported and not done by the laboratory. I questioned and had to renegotiate remuneration of pathologists and radiologists, all with knowledge of the president of the board, and I have done nothing without involving the medical executive committee. . . .

As far as nursing goes, here is a list of what I have done: I have met with all shifts, with head nurses, with supervisors, and regularly with the director and assistant directors. I hired a new director and fired an old assistant director whom the nurses said showed favoritism, lied to them, and overpromised. . . . I hired an expert nursing consultant to help us develop appropriate goals and ways of meeting these goals. I was in the process of obtaining the services of an operations research consultant, at no cost to the hospital, to help us with our scheduling problems. We implemented a study done by an administrative resident on improved staffing and scheduling. I pointed out all the problems of authoritarian leadership, lack of adequate quality assurance programs, and lack of appropriate scheduling and budgeting to the previous nursing director, which is why she had to be demoted. . . .

I could go through each of the charges made by the people assembled here, but it won't really prove anything. Yes, I did call a doctor a sonofabitch in my office. Yes, I did leave the hospital after the bomb scare before the police came, but only after I was convinced that it was a scare. I had a meeting to go to in the city, and I called one hour later to see that everything was all right. I think it is significant that none of the department heads supposedly humiliated by me showed up at this meeting. You have asked me to resign, but I'm not going to resign. That would not solve the hospital's problems. Firing me will not solve the bad nursing morale here or the doctor mistrust. It will show the doctors and nurses and the community who runs this hospital. Is it the board of trustees or some doctors and nurses (the nurses are mainly being used by the doctors)? Whose head will these doctors be asking for the next time they want to get rid of somebody? The bond issue set for next month that could refinance our debt on the new wing will not go through if you fire me. And we shall have a $355,000 payment to make in August which will be difficult to meet. (Kovner, 1997)

A vote was taken to clear me of the charges without rebuttal, and this passed seven in favor, five against, with four abstentions. Later, the board voted unanimously to dismiss me with two months' severance, after a ten to six vote to fire me.

Moral of the Story

In retrospect, I believe that I had made the mistake of taking the board of trustees literally when members told me that my job was to improve quality and contain costs (and to improve access to medical care for the community if financially feasible). Also, I was an outsider, and these were medical and nursing professionals many of whom had grown up together and who had certainly worked together at Anytown for years.

The board chair supported me until the end, and our failure was certainly a great disappointment to him. His good intentions had been severely punished by doctors and nurses, many of whom he knew socially. One board member said that whether I was right or wrong, the doctors didn't like me and I should have fired the associate administrator and the director of nursing who were submarining me from the start. Another said that although he thought I could do an excellent job managing a university hospital, I definitely couldn't do the job at this hospital, and they should have gotten rid of me now.

In retrospect, I probably shouldn't have taken the job. If I wanted to be a manager, I should have looked for and accepted a more modest job, perhaps in a university hospital, back home in New York City, as an assistant or associate director. My firing had large personal costs—mostly in stress to our marriage, but professionally the job loss turned out not to be too serious a setback.

Lessons Learned in Anytown About Health Care Delivery

I believe it makes sense to: (1) cover all Americans for national health insurance, with minimum benefits a la Medicare; (2) force accountability by those purchasing care for large populations, as some employers do in negotiating with health plans (and as some health plans do in negotiating with doctors and hospitals); and, (3) close many hospitals, and use the money in ways that are more cost effective for improving health of populations.

In Anytown, I learned a great deal about the role of a hospital in its community. The United States has a lot more hospitals and hospital beds than it needs. Hospitals operate at less than 60% of capacity nationwide. In the Anytown area, one hospital could have sufficed for three communities. Today, in many communities hospital mergers are taking place. Hospitals are merging largely for financial reasons, often with little change over the short run, other than they have greater bargaining power in contracting with managed care companies. Boards want independent hospitals so they can remain as board members. Doctors want independent hospitals so that their autonomy can be maximized. Nonprofit hospitals are not effectively accountable to those who pay for hospital care. But to what extent are independent small hospitals in the interests of patients and taxpayers?

Patients do not generally pay much of their own hospital bills, as health insurance is purchased by employers. Taxpayers don't see their taxes going to pay to support nonprofit hospitals; the taxes these hospitals don't pay on their property or income bears little relationship to the taxes any individual pays. Communities such as Anytown have a fair amount of local pride in "our" hospital, "our" doctors, "our" trustees, when the hospital is not part of a large national corporation, and is in "our" town to stay.

HMOs and managed care plans have been invented partly to cure the accountability problem. The plan gets a fixed amount of money for a defined package of benefits and then negotiates with hospitals and doctors to keep costs down yet assure acceptable quality. Employers negotiate with health plans who compete with each other. Some attending physicians make their living primarily from the hospital, and yet are either in competition with the hospital, like some orthopedists in sports medicine, or have conflicting interests, as, for example, some cardiologists who have had sweetheart economic deals with hospitals to interpret ECGs, which can be scanned more or less equally well, and more cheaply, tele-mechanically.

I think it's comparatively more cost effective to spend health dollars on initiatives that involve helping persons to lead healthier lives, or spending money to help community organizations (of which the hospital is one), to accomplish this. For example, churches can be funded to establish buddy systems to transport young mothers-to-be who need prenatal care. However, such access to care is not first priority for many Americans who are primarily concerned with their own health. Moreover, hospital boards, such as Anytown's, want to raise money for new diagnostic equipment which will help physicians augment their incomes rather than to get low income persons access to primary care. This is reflected in comments such as, *"They should have to work for a living like we do in which case they can afford decent health care, which costs me a lot of money. And we certainly don't want the government running everything."*

At Anytown, I was involved in moving the board's agenda, as I understood it. Obviously, I had no power in Anytown to influence national health insurance and was fully occupied trying to run a medium-sized hospital. I tried to move the hospital in the direction of providing higher quality care at a more reasonable cost and with more adequate access, but this wasn't what my employers were really paying me to do. (They were paying me to serve the doctors in their private practice.) None of the local hospitals was going to close or merge voluntarily, and then only on terms most favorable to them.

Lessons Learned at Anytown Hospital About Management

Written with the benefit of hindsight, it is better for managers not to say what they are thinking, but to say rather what they think other people want them to say. I'm not speaking here about giving up or giving in regarding principles. Only I would like to suggest, however, that there is a way of speaking about things and a way not to speak about things. I would encourage any manager to pay attention to timing and questions of tone. I would also encourage any manager to carefully analyze the community in which he or she will manage and come up with an appropriate strategy for living there.

I learned about the importance of hearing what people are *not* saying when they are talking to you. People are generally very careful about what they *do* say, but they leave out what it is they think you don't want to hear. People are not going to tell you that you are sarcastic or arrogant, only that you are pretty smart. People are going to tell you about how good your ideas are, not that Doctor Jones' nose was bent out of shape when you contradicted him in front of some other doctors, especially since you were right about the point in question. Most importantly, the board of Anytown Hospital was telling me, yes improve or try to improve the quality of care and contain costs, so long as you don't get the physicians sufficiently upset that they think they have to organize to get rid of you, and replace you with some other administrator whom they can trust and who will understand what the game he is being well paid for really is about. This game is not to upset the apple cart, although it's fine to talk about how tasty the apples are and are going to be. No one ever questioned my motivations or even the soundness of my ideas; it was more that my persona didn't fit in here, and my ideas, at least how I expressed them, weren't appropriate for this place at this time.

Reflection: On Appraising Performance

As Charles Handy (1998) has suggested, most institutional appraisal systems end up by "damaging morale and changing nothing" (p. 128). Part of the reason is that appraisals are formally done and only once a year, usually in relation to pay raises. Think of the following situations for boss Charlie Pierce who must appraise these three employees:

1. Sol Fries is a low performer. Pierce is afraid that if he appraises Fries accurately, Fries will either withdraw still further at work or pursue another job. Meanwhile Pierce believes it is better to have Fries at current productivity than to have no one and carry out still another search.

2. Estelle Clark is a high performer. She was brought in at a low salary and deserves a higher raise than what Pierce is going to recommend (although the raise is above average). Estelle does not function well, however, without constant support and close supervision. Estelle is extremely sensitive to criticism, even if this is constructive, which is why Pierce doesn't say anything "negative" to her.

3. Tyrone Biggs is a high performer. He complains that he doesn't get the information that he needs to do his job and about the incredible bureaucratic hurdles to accomplish or launch anything significant. He

also feels "alone" or "exposed" on any assignment which involves risk; and that blame for failure will be assigned to Tyrone while credit for success will go to someone else.

Perhaps these examples tell us more about Charlie Pierce, as an evaluator, than about difficulties in appraising performance. Of course, appraising performance isn't difficult to do if objectives and strategies are negotiated in advance with a relevant employee, and communication between appraiser and appraisee about performance occurs regularly, with objectives and strategies being changed and adapted over time as appropriate. Another good idea is for every manager to develop her own learning objectives, outside of the objectives for her regular work; and for every boss to specify in advance development objectives for those managers he supervises. Now why doesn't this happen more often in health care organizations?

The usual explanations are that the supervising managers don't see it in their interest to change their own behavior. If there are no incentives to change behavior, why should they rock the boat? It is only when limits of organizational performance are not met that scapegoats must be found.

There are two implications for the aspiring health care manager who wants to improve performance and improve appraising performance. First, invest a lot of time in job searches. You want to work for a boss who will take an interest in your development and for an organization that is growing or succeeding in the marketplace. Second, as Tom Peters (1997, p. 186) says, "think resume." Can you work up a resume/curriculum vitae each year that is noticeably/discernably/distinctly different from what it would have been the previous year? Review with your boss and subordinates just how you are going to accomplish this, what you want and expect from them, ask them if they have any problems with what you want and expect. With the key persons you supervise, meet with them off premises, explain to them what you want, negotiate with them what you will expect to see by the end of the year, follow it up in writing, ask if there is any other way you can help them so that they can achieve what it was you agreed that they were going to achieve.

Nobody wants to get fired, but if you are going to be fired, this should be on your own terms. You should be able to see it coming, and it should occur amicably, or at least impersonally. Leaving may reasonably often be viewed to have certain advantages for both parties. This kind of understanding is what you want to achieve with persons whom you have to let go as well. The appraiser and the appraisee disagree as to what the appraisee is or was to accomplish. Or they differ as to how the work will be or was accomplished. Someone has to leave, and the appraiser's boss has agreed with the appraiser that this is going to be the appraisee. Could this have been avoided by in-depth conversation at the beginning?

Appraising Performance: A Checklist

Yes	No	
_____	_____	Have you appraised your performance recently?
_____	_____	Did your appraisal largely agree with that of the person who appraised you?
_____	_____	Are you satisfied with the way you appraise those who work for you?
_____	_____	Can you think of ways to improve the appraisal process?
_____	_____	Do you have learning objectives for the next 12 months?
_____	_____	Is your resume distinctly better than it was 12 months ago?
_____	_____	Do you know now what your next job is likely to be?
_____	_____	Do you know what skills and experience are required that you need to improve in order to increase your chances of landing that job?

Practical Exercise

Write a paper on your career objectives and how you plan to achieve them. Discuss your current experience in terms of managerial roles, skills, and values. Specify a desired job you wish to get within 3–5 years and indicate the skills and experience required to obtain and excel in the desired job. Indicate how you are going to get from where you are to where you want to be. Discuss any constraints to implementation and how these can be overcome. Review your plan with peers and mentors.

7

Consultant to Large Foundations

I have never worked as a full-time salaried employee for a large philan-
thropic foundation, but I have spent 14 years, from 1981 through 1994,
working as program director or co-program director for four large demonstration (pilot) programs, funded by The Robert Wood Johnson Foundation
(RWJ), in Princeton, NJ, and the W.K. Kellogg Foundation, in Battle
Creek, MI. These were 25%–40% time job commitments, while I was
otherwise employed as a full-time faculty member at the Robert F.
Wagner Graduate School of Public Service, at New York University, in
New York City. My research in management and governance in health
care has also been funded by the Commonwealth Foundation in New
York City and by the Pew Charitable Trusts, in Philadelphia, PA.

The Rural Hospital Program of Extended Care Services for Johnson,
spanning 1981–1986 was the first demonstration program that I directed, and in many ways the most successful. I was recommended to Bob
Blendon, then a senior official of RWJ, by a former student of mine at
the Wharton School, Chris Grant, who was then working for Blendon.
At Johnson, staff had developed the new program, and were looking for
someone to run it. I was, on the face of it, a logical choice, as I had managed a rural hospital, and nursing home. Since I was then an academic (at
NYU), I had the time to do the work.

At that time, The Robert Wood Johnson Foundation had assets
approaching $1 billion, and RWJ spent about half of their distributions
each year running 10–20 large national demonstration programs. As Bob
Blendon explained to me, the idea behind Johnson's staffing approach
was not to run national programs directly out of the foundation. They
wished to avoid permanent commitments to specific programs. Rather,
replicative programs were to funded by others. Each national program

had an evaluation component, which was separately funded and administered. Thus, each national program director related to three sets of RWJ staff–program, finance, and evaluation, as well as to the evaluation director, usually a faculty member at another university. Most demonstration programs were advised by a national committee and oversaw grants at up to 25 sites.

There was great chemistry between Bob Blendon and me. Bob had wonderful ideas, sparkling wit, and incredible energy. He was also my idea of a gentleman. One of the best things about working with the Johnson Foundation staff for me was that it allowed me to be a gentleman. In other words, it allowed me to do things based on the merits, without undue responsiveness to provider interests. The big hurdle I had to jump to get this assignment (most of the national programs were directed by physicians) was being approved by David Rogers, MD, then president of the foundation. Blendon asked me to get references, preferably from physicians, and I was fortunate to know and be known by two physicians within Dr. Rogers' circle, both, as he was, doctors of internal medicine. These were Sam Thier, who was then chief of Medicine at Yale, and Sam Martin, a stalwart in the graduate programs in medicine and business at the University of Pennsylvania. (I have never forgotten Sam Martin's description of a manager in a difficult situation as "having as much chance as a one-legged man in an ass-kicking contest.") So our interview was low-key. Dr. Rogers wanted to know that he could trust me, looking to Bob Blendon for assurance that I was competent to carry out the work.

As so often happens, the success of this demonstration program was largely beyond our control and rested on the willingness of the federal government to pay for short-term, long-term care ("swing beds") in small rural hospitals. In this way hospitals could use otherwise vacant beds to provide long-term care to patients, thus avoiding some nursing home transfers and easing others. The program was vigorously opposed by the nursing home industry as a "foot in the door" to hospitals taking over part of their domain. The program had been enacted with the support of the small, rural hospitals and funded as part of Medicare, but at that point in time, prior to the commencement of the RWJ program, the details of Medicare payment were not yet worked out. This caused us some anxious moments, but after the regulations were approved, it was pretty much clear sailing.

This demonstration program was divided into two phases. First, Johnson provided funding to state hospital associations to assist them in developing capabilities for technical assistance and education which they would provide to the small rural hospitals. State hospital associations selected to participate were in Kansas, Mississippi, Missouri, New Mexico, and North Dakota. In the demonstration's second phase, 26 small rural hospitals in these five states were selected to develop models of swing-bed services. The state hospital associations assisted these grantee hospitals and other eligible hospitals in their respective states in developing high quality extended care services to meet the special needs of the elderly, in instituting an internal quality assurance process, and, in strengthening financial management and third-party reimbursement. The job of the program office was to help make sure that everything was happening as it should, while the financial arm of the foundation audited the grantees' books, and the formal evaluators made their reports after the project was completed. The program office had three full-time staff besides myself— Hila Richardson, who was the associate program director, a program assistant, and a secretary. Our National Advisory Council chaired by Rheba DeTorynay, nursing school dean at the University of Washington, met annually.

We found that the hospital association could play an important role in providing technical assistance and in overcoming problems in state level regulatory certification and reimbursement. While the swing-bed program, could not, on its own, save a failing hospital, it could provide revenue to help a hospital survive. The program provided effective and appropriate care for some patients and swing beds often functioned as a springboard to other areas of diversification and could help small rural hospitals move out of their traditional, acute care role.

Lessons Learned from Swing Beds

The Robert Wood Johnson Foundation ran an impressive and well-financed program, which I appreciated, given my previous experience. This did not entail spending a lot of money, but rather having sufficient funds so that everything that should be done was done (within the parameters of available funding and RWJ rules and operating procedures). The programmatic or project focus was protected (after funds had been allocated) from financial constraints and interventions from outside the program.[1]

Through working with RWJ, I learned about how a large foundation functions and about how large national demonstrations are run. Large foundations operate as bureaucracies, and, similar to my experience with

---

[1] Budgets are often adjusted ex post facto in health care organizations.

the UAW in dealing with Michigan Blue Cross, I had to learn how to get things done at the foundation. This meant, occasionally, not going through the usual channels. I could have gone to Bob Blendon, but I chose not to bog him down with the details. Generally speaking, changes could be made through the designated program officer, and I was fortunate to have several good ones, demonstrating again how important personal relationships are. In part, my good relations in the swing-bed program were based on the underlying trust and confidence of Bob Blendon, and through him, Dave Rogers.

Through operating the rural health program I learned a great deal about rural hospitals and about rural America. I spent a lot of time flying over and driving in vast, sparsely populated rural areas. We would alight in small rural communities where the hospital was often the principal employer, and on a good day, had from 15 to 20 patients. Such hospitals were usually run very efficiently, typically on a less costly basis than larger urban hospitals. This was because economies of scale did not pertain in these hospitals. For example, they staffed their units with nurses who were called in and paid by the hour (they were nonunionized) rather than by the day or by the week. When more specialized medical services were required, they were provided by teams who flew in from larger cities for one afternoon a week or a month to a small hospital in Mississippi or North Dakota. A final lesson was learning how to get some kind of a successor program funded by the foundation, as I was having so much fun and learning so much in running this program.

The Hospital-Based Rural Health Care Program

I succeeded in getting a successor, the Hospital-Based Rural Health Care Program, funded by RWJ. Its goals were to strengthen the ability of rural hospitals to provide a high quality of care and to promote the financial stability of these institutions. For these purposes, the foundation provided four-year grants averaging $600,000 each to as many as 15 groups of hospitals and other health care organizations serving rural areas. In addition, a total of up to $7.5 million in loans was made available to grantees to upgrade or expand their service capacity, up to $500,000 for each grantee.

The program sought to support consortia of hospitals and related providers in their implementation of any or all of the following strategies:

- *Improving organizational arrangements* by forming linkages among hospitals and other providers through regionalization or affiliation.

- *Promoting cost-efficiency through improved management* by sharing data and billing systems, management teams, the purchase of supplies and new technology, and the recruitment and employment of physicians and specialized staff.
- *Expanding revenue bases* by diversifying into new health and health-related services (e.g., long-term care); improving the quality and delivery of currently provided services; developing joint ventures, forming capitated systems, and expanding utilization for existing services.

Our National Advisory Council was a diverse group of experts, chaired by Dr. Christopher Fordham, chancellor of the University of North Carolina at Chapel Hill. The program director interacted with RWJ program officers, financial and evaluation officers, and evaluators from the University of Minnesota. Over 400 letters of intent were received from hospitals in 48 states. One-hundred-eighty applications representing 33 states were reviewed. Thirteen grants were awarded to consortia representing 182 rural hospitals in 12 states.

An example of the program in action was the technical assistance programs being implemented by the Rural Wisconsin Hospital Cooperative. Their financial management program coordinated meetings among the consortia members' financial officers. They discussed common concerns, problem-solving techniques, and new legislation, implementing a "benchmarking" process to identify and replicate best practices, in areas such as billing patients. The exchange of ideas resulted in improved Medicare reimbursements, cash flows, and operating cost margins. Programs conducted by RWJ-funded consortia included recruitment and retention of clinicians in Montana, acute bed conversion and loans for ambulatory care facilities in North Carolina, shared clinical and referral services in Upstate New York, and technical assistance for quality improvement, again in Wisconsin.

The "rural hospital" program was not as successful as "swing beds" for a variety of reasons. Although there are many ways of measuring success, here, I measure success by examining whether or not what was demonstrated showed enough promise that it was picked up and replicated by many other organizations. A measure of lack of success would be its demonstration as a failure—thus other replications would *not* be attempted. Neither the consortium idea nor the funding of such consortia directly followed, so far as we knew.

I think the major stumbling block in making demonstration programs work is management or "implementation." Implementation is typically carried out by managers. And the managers of the small, rural hospitals which received the grants can be characterized as not very long in the job, or as not very well-trained for the job. In general, the board members of these small, nonprofit hospitals lacked both the skills and experience to guide the formulation of goals and strategies or to evaluate top management. The foundation has had a bias against funding support for management as an integral part of health care. Perhaps the RWJ board associates management with large for-profit corporations, whose activities they don't wish to support.

During the life of this demonstration, the leadership at RWJ changed. David Rogers resigned, reportedly around issues relative to his power relative to that of the board, and Bob Blendon left too, to begin a new career in polling relative to public policy, as a Harvard professor. After this change in management, I experienced personal differences with my new program officer and, when the grant had ended, stopped working for RWJ.

Under its new leadership, RWJ moved away from national demonstrations, as they felt that they could achieve more for less by spending their immense funds in other ways. RWJ pays more attention now to charting "natural" demonstrations, rather than devising and carrying out the demonstrations with affiliated University partners. I remain convinced that health care delivery needs more demonstrations, experimentation, and evaluative research, and that demonstrations often require outside funding.

The Advanced Management Program for Clinicians

The W. K. Kellogg Foundation, like RWJ, is one of the nation's largest foundations, giving away tens of millions of dollars annually. Unlike RWJ, which is health based and U.S.-restricted, Kellogg gives large sums of monies also to sectors other than health care, such as agriculture, education, and community development, as well as to health care, in the United States and around the world. Three main differences existed between Kellogg and RWJ in administration. First, there was a lack of hands-on oversight at Kellogg, which leaves administration in the hands of the program director. Second, Kellogg lacked a program of large outside evaluation of demonstrations. Third, there was no money in Kellogg program budgets for overhead. At Kellogg, I worked closely with Bob DeVries, Kellogg's chief program officer for health care. My codirector for the Advanced Management Program for Clinicians (AMPC) at NYU was Professor Victor Rodwin, who is an expert in comparative health systems.

The grant was submitted in August 1985. Victor and I proposed to establish an interdisciplinary advanced training program for health care professionals who sought management responsibilities and leadership positions, those who already had management responsibilities as well as those who sought to make career shifts in this direction. Since the clinicians we sought to attract came from diverse backgrounds and had a range of professional goals, we felt it was essential not to impose a formulaic approach in the design of curriculum.

For candidates seeking a Master of Science degree in management or policy, we allowed a choice of six courses, to be selected by individual participants in conjunction with their advisor. The full resources of New York University were available to all participants. These included courses in the schools of law, business, medicine, social work, arts and sciences, and education (in which NYU's nursing program is located). We required only three required courses in this individually tailored curriculum; both semesters of the year-long Kellogg seminar in health policy and management, and a course of independent study, culminating in a final paper. Clinicians who already had advanced degrees and no particular interest in obtaining further degrees could obtain an Advanced Professional Certificate by completing five courses in one area of specialization. Those clinicians who simply wanted to take a course or two were occasionally accepted as special students and invited to participate in the AMPC program.

The Kellogg seminar played an integrating role in each clinician's individually tailored program of study. The seminar exposed them to the literature in the field, stimulated discussion and analysis of issues, introduced them to the program's faculty and to leaders in the field, and developed a group esprit de corps. Seminar themes included the health care industry's current structure and evolution, shifts in federal and state policies and the implications for clinicians and managers, and the response by managers in health care organizations to change.

Since most AMPC participants held full-time jobs, we converted the final paper into a pragmatic, professional project, that took one of two forms. It could result in a case study (several of which were subsequently published in a casebook I edited with David Kindig, 1992) complete with a teaching note based on an analysis of management problems or policy issues affecting health care organizations, or it could result in a paper that began by the clinician identifying a problem in some health care organization, and then reviewing the literature, comparing how other similar organizations have dealt with similar challenges. Under either option, the final paper always involved individual attention to each participant's project by two members of NYUs's core faculty. This process often sparked in the clinician a new interest in the literature, methods, and theories current in the field that were often shared among participants, lecturers, and faculty.

Kellogg mainly funded fellowships for clinicians, but also program development, marketing, and administration. The program (a 3-year grant of $375,000) was small, with a planned matriculation of 20 participants each year by the end of year three (a goal which we achieved). Although roughly three-fourths of the first 90 AMPC clinicians were physicians, the program was originally conceived (as Kellogg insisted) for a broad range of clinicians, including dentists, nurses, and social workers. We felt it was important to expose AMPC participants to a multidisciplinary approach (since this was the nature of the challenges they had to meet in practice), and to link the program, through the use of case studies and guest lecturers, with clinician faculty, management practitioners, and policy makers. We thus formed an inter-school committee of affiliated NYU faculty to tap some of the leading scholars in other schools at NYU and to improve linkages with schools and practitioners.

The program was immensely successful for the Wagner School of NYU, where the program was self-financed after the Kellogg grant ended. The program enriched the quality of our regular classes, as AMPC participants took our normal classes with students pursing the MPA or PhD degree. In part as a result of our success, Kellogg funded at least one program at another university for physician managers, and other schools started similar educational programs. Although NYU's program has been physician-dominated, it has not been exclusively for physicians. Kellogg funding allowed clinicians the chance to attend such a program. The program has helped many clinicians in obtaining managerial positions.

The program, however, has had a number of issues, most of which centered around clinicians. There were three major questions. First, do clinicians trained in management require courses different from those being taken by other Masters' students in health care policy and management? Second, to what extent should Wagner encourage clinicians to pursue management training when they will be competing for jobs with our other graduates? Third, for the clinicians, when does it and does it not make sense to seek what kinds of management training?

My position on these issues follows. We found that although clinicians obtaining management education do not require courses different from those that our other students take (many of whom are clinicians), Wagner must develop courses in addition to those we regularly offer, to better serve our clinician students. As of 1998, such courses included medical management (to include utilization management, disease management, and population health) professional ethics, and nonprofit entrepreneurship.

Such courses would benefit all Wagner students. We decided to encourage clinicians with management jobs to seek training in the skills and experience they require to do such jobs effectively, and to educate clinicians similarly who want such jobs, whether or not such jobs are also desired by program graduates who are not clinicians. The lack of success as a practitioner is not a sufficient reason to become a manager. Rather, an interested clinician should be someone who enjoys managing and has the temperament to enjoy being a manager. This means being able to get people to work together to achieve common goals when managers lack the power to be able to tell people "what to do or else." Managers learn how to be comfortable with ambiguity, deal with people who are not saying what they mean, and make decisions absent all the necessary data. Many scientists do not have this kind of inclination or preference. Some clinicians, however, have strengths as managers: They are smart, action oriented, and data driven. I greatly enjoyed developing the AMPC program, working with Victor Rodwin and Bob DeVries and with the clinician participants, and showing the results that we were able to achieve.

The Hospital Community Benefit Standards Program

The most promising demonstration I was ever involved in was the brainchild of one of the most unforgettable people I have ever met, Bob Sigmond. As Bob Sigmond stated in our 1988 grant proposal, standards have never been developed for community hospitals relating explicitly to community benefit or community service. Existing hospital standards did not address issues relating to the community's health status, or to the cost, quality, relevance, redundancy, and accessibility of the community's health services. As a result hospitals are more likely to be viewed as part of the contemporaneous health service problems, rather than as important parts of potential solutions. We proposed a demonstration involving the development and testing of highly credible, feasible community benefit standards at 24 hospitals, leading to an ongoing, self-financed, certification program. Such a program, we believed, could serve in the same way that the accreditation program of the Joint Commission on Accreditation of Health Care Organizations has in the past, as a badge of contemporary excellence for those wishing to identify the most ethical institutions.

In the proposal, we added that the major forces acting on hospitals had the effect of diverting energies from concern about the health status of people in the community and the cost and accessibility of their health care service, (as contrasted with the financial well-being of the hospital and the quality of its products). While providers did not actively oppose the concept of community benefit, such an ideal was very difficult to implement without some clear cut sense of direction. We sought to implement community benefit standards, as set forth in a manner that could be understood and supported—not only by hospital and medical leadership, but also by community leaders and by funders.

Such standards, we believed, had to be explicit enough that the hospital's successes and failures in their efforts to benefit the community could be clearly identified, yet flexible enough to be adapted to a wide variety of community environments as well as to varying amounts and kinds of individual hospital resources and skills. Any voluntary hospital should be able to achieve the standards, but they should be more demanding than regulatory requirements that might be administered by governmental agencies responsible for hospital licensing and tax-exemption decisions.

We formed an extraordinary national steering committee. Bob became the committee chair, and other members included Ed Connors, president of Mercy Health Services in Michigan, Jane Delgado, Chief Executive of the National Coalition of Hispanic Health and Human Service Organizations in Washington DC, Paul Hofmann, executive vice president of Alta Bates Corporation, in California, Sam Thier, president of the Institute of Medicine in Washington DC, and Bruce Vladeck, president of the United Hospital Fund, in New York. Bob recruited Paul Hattis as full-time deputy director. Both a physician and a lawyer, he worked at the time in the legal department of the American Hospital Association.

After a great deal of work and after receiving a great deal of advice, we then invited community hospitals in the United States to participate in the Hospital Community Benefit Standards Program (HCBSP). Then we sought to demonstrate the value of a systematic approach to community service, in accordance with national standards. These new standards, developed by the program's national steering committee, were based on the community service policy positions of the American Hospital Association and the American College of Healthcare Executives. These standards called for a disciplined, management approach to community benefit objectives, similar to the approach required of hospitals by certification programs related to patient care quality assurance, infection control, medical and nursing education, and all other activities.

And so, the HCBSP developed four standards for hospitals to attain, each followed by a number of required characteristics. The standards were as follows:

• Evidence of the hospital's formal commitment to a community benefit program for a designated community.

• The scope of the program includes hospital-sponsored projects for the designated community in each of the following areas: improving health status, addressing the health problems of minorities, the poor and other medically underserved populations, and containing the growth of community health care costs.

• The hospital's program includes activities designed to stimulate other organizations and individuals to join in carrying out a broad health agenda in the designated community.

• The hospital fosters an internal environment that encourages hospital wide involvement in the program.

Under the program, demonstration hospitals did not receive any money for their pioneering efforts. They would receive technical assistance and advice to support their efforts to make the necessary changes to meet the standards. They also would be likely to receive much public attention and support for their efforts.

During the winter of 1991 and the spring of 1992, the HCBSP surveyed what became the 49 demonstration hospitals and received 34 responses which indicated: (1) some major gains in hospital commitment to reforming health care in their designated communities; (2) development of new projects and shaping of existing projects; (3) moving significantly toward developing collaborative agendas with community leaders and in focusing on populations; and, (4) varying involvement among different constituencies in HCBSP hospitals. In 1992, HCBSP transitioned from NYU to the American Hospital Association which was to work on designing a collaborative community benefit agenda as part of its health reform strategy.

After we had transitioned the grant I interviewed Bob as to what we had done "right" and "wrong" about HCBSP. He suggested that we had done the following things "right." We stayed away from the tax exemption question for nonprofit institutions. We based our program on AHA guidelines. We rooted our notion of community benefit programming in modern management, that is, a hospital could shape up a quite credible community benefit program by simply managing existing resources and relationships more systematically (lack of management rather than lack of resources or lack of commitment being the real problem, at least in the initial phase). We stayed with the long-range goal of demonstrating that community benefit programming is an essential element of health care reform. We selected and worked with an unusually dedicated group of demonstration hospitals. We transitioned the program to the AHA. We were right to be flexible and change direction, as circumstances indicated, for example, giving up our notion of building standards into the JCAHO program (JCAHO had very different priorities). We had to give up on hospital conformance with standards as the key measure of our success and on our original goal of turning our program over to some other organization as a self-supporting activity. We held inflexibly to two key concepts: the notion of the power of voluntary standards as a key force in stimulating better behavior in the health field; and, rooting health care reform in community benefit, not simply the unseen hand of the market and governmental police power, important as they were.

Bob suggested that HCBSP had done the following things "wrong." We stayed too long with the JCAHO concept and with the notion of conformance to standards rather than standards as guidelines, and we selected too many demonstration hospitals, when we couldn't give each one of them sufficient attention. We didn't devote enough energy to making sure that our demonstration hospitals and others were really committed to the concept of community and community benefits in health care reform, and we didn't devote enough time and energy in articulating these notions. We didn't realize until too late that a university setting with part-time staff wasn't the right setting for any business development activity on a national level. In retrospect, Bob would have focused more on the role of the hospital as a community institution in the development of community care networks, addressing the vision of health care reform through the evolution of community care networks (Kovner, 1994a).

Lessons Learned from HCBSP

As a consultant, I again realized the importance of effective management in operating hospital community benefit programs around the country. Indeed, a hospital can shape up a quite credible community benefit program by simply managing existing resources and relationships more systematically, as Sigmond has argued. The key here is to specify the current circumstances in sufficient detail, identifying the related problems and issues of concern, before envisioning changes in those activities.

In analyzing our own office what I find astonishing is that we accomplished as much as we did, given the differing expectations and goals of the three leading participants—Bob Sigmond, Paul Hattis, and me. (The situation reminds me of the three ancient Romans, Augustus, Marc

Antony, and Lepidus, briefly sharing power after Caesar's murder.) Three is an unhappy number to share governance, as two will almost always gang up against one. HCBSP was Bob's program, and yet since this was a NYU grant I had to be the program director. We had differences over the allocation of grant resources and other issues.

My comments as guest editor for a special issue of *The Journal of Health Administration Education* on "Community Benefit Programs for Health Care Organizations" demonstrate my views. In my editorial, I suggested that community care networks are a response which should be given more attention by policy makers to improve Americans' health status and access to care and to contain increases in health care costs. I responded to devil's advocate questions: "What is community, anyway?" "Why isn't providing health care to HMO enrollees, without regard to community initiatives, the best way of organizing health services? Why do we need community care networks; why don't we have them anyway (Kovner, 1994b)?

Bob Sigmond's opinions are also of note here. His primary point was that most health care (aside from group practice HMOs) has been organized primarily to serve individual, sick patients, rather than primarily to serve populations. Obviously, serving sick patients is quite different from organizing to serve populations of mostly well people. Community approaches can better address problems such as AIDS and other chronic illnesses and disabilities, teenage pregnancy, violence, drug abuse, health promotion and disease prevention, among others. Economies can be achieved from initiatives at the community level, where people live. Lifestyle is significantly influenced by how the community is organized. Sigmond concluded that capitation payment to health services organizations combined with much more systematic management of broadened community benefit incentives would facilitate movement in the direction of integrating care of patients, populations, and communities. While I agree with Bob's theoretical arguments on community health, in practice, an efficient population for a large health care organization to effectively serve is probably about 300,000. This population in many areas comprises many communities. Yet, in my own case, I do not feel a part of any specific community. Neither my geographic neighborhood, apartment complex, university, or apartment floor feels like a community.

While I think that Sigmond is correct regarding the contribution of community organization to improving the health status of a community, and believe that it is more efficient to do regional planning from a geographic perspective, I am not convinced of its efficacy in most of this country. This is largely based on personal experience in settings as diverse as suburban Detroit, or in center city Philadelphia. It could work in a place like Anytown, but what I remember so distinctly about Anytown were the rival "patronage and boycott" groups, to use Freidson's (1972, p. 193) term, among people who didn't want many neighbors in their group, church or "community."

Consumers want health care on a commodity basis, for a specific illness or a diagnosis, not as a life-time purchase as part of a formal planning process. Maybe lifetime health status and goals are what people should want, but they don't appear to want them. Health care organizations located in geographic proximity should certainly work together, and they should work together with community organizations that can affect the health of a population. This is different from capitating local health budgets and then allocating the resources locally as part of a political process. Providers working together are good for people's health care and good for business. This can translate into improved health status for consumers and improved productivity in health care provision. Certainly those who use health care organizations should have a voice in how they operate or be afforded an exit in the form of access to services provided by competitors.

The HCBSP program focused and clarified my previous ideas regarding the proper role of government in health care. I believe that it is important that local or regional health departments set standards, evaluate how local providers meet or do not meet the standards, and influence local consumers and taxpayers to allocate local resources appropriately. These ideas are no doubt as quixotic as Bob's regarding community benefit incentives. But I believe strongly in getting government out of the direct provision of health services, as government cannot effectively hold itself accountable for such delivery. Rather, government should hold the private sector accountable. This suggestion is realistic, given the current politics of the United States, and this is aligned with the political interests of many in the legislative and executive branches of government and with the interests of most providers.

HCBSP focused attention on the central problem of nonprofit organizations, which is their lack of accountability. Government officials are replaceable by voters, as are for-profit CEOs by shareholders. Nonprofit boards are usually accountable only to themselves, and many of these boards do not even try to do a good job of sharing information as to what they intend to do as a board and as an organization with relevant stakeholders. Nor do they actually disclose how organizational performance during a past year measures up to how they said the organization was going to perform, giving reasons to stakeholders for why performance met or didn't meet expectations and why performance or objectives or both need to be changed and how for the next year.

Two Program Ideas

Two of my more recent ideas that I hope to get funded from large foundations are the following: a formal analysis of health insurance and an examination of typical board practices and their use of information. The first idea would involve a formal analysis of various suggestions regarding national health insurance. What are the main leading approaches for national health insurance, such as either extending Medicare or Medicaid managed care to the whole population? What are their pros and cons? Who are the winners and losers under the present system of health care financing? What are the problems and issues raised by the present system? How could we get a better system without spending any more money? What is known about some of the key issues, and what needs to be studied? I would like to put these issues into sensible, practical language, circulate these findings to various interest groups, note their comments, and share this information with the public.

My second idea would examine typical board practices with regard to the information management provides them to make decisions. I would compare this with best practice (high performing) boards who obtain information, for example, on employee, physician, patient's (and nonuser) expectations and perceptions regarding quality and service, as well as on the usual financial indicators. How should this information be most usefully presented to the board? Also, what information should boards regularly get regarding the strengths and weaknesses of competitors, or about how quality and service processes in their organization compare with those of benchmark leading providers?

Reflection: Working with Foundations

As Ernest Hemingway has said in *The Snows of Kilimanjaro* (1936) *the difference between the rich and the rest of us is that the rich have more money.* This brings me to the topics of foundations, funders, philanthropists, and inspiring the confidence of those with money to invest in the mission of health care delivery programs. Consider these situations:

1. Pat Quinones works for a struggling neighborhood health center in downtown Detroit, and tries to raise money from foundations for worthy programs. She regularly receives nicely written turndowns on fine stationery, which inform her that what she is requesting is not currently among that foundation's priorities.

2. Sam Bailey has received a large foundation grant to help combat violence in the inner cities. He in turn must "ride herd" over 15 local grantees all of whom want to spend money for certain line items, such as local transportation for clients that foundation officials say does not comply with their rules. The local grantees insist that other foundation officials had previously told them otherwise. Sam also doesn't agree with the methods being used by foundation-funded evaluators measuring program success.

3. Clara Gold is administrative assistant to the executive director of a foundation to prevent child abuse. The 90-year-old board chair has been in office for 40 years and the current board members neither help plan the foundation's future, raise money, nor evaluate the executive director. Clara believes that the executive director is content with things the way that they are, although Clara was recruited explicitly to help "turn things around."

Some health care managers wish to become president of a small foundation. Many of our NYU students work in foundations. I have had only positive experiences in receiving several large grants from a small number of foundations and in working with some capable foundation officials driven by a sense of mission. Yet, the world of foundations is a bit removed from most people's reality. Each foundation has its own history, culture, and politics, much of which is quite different from that of local health care delivery organizations.

So how do you get a large foundation grant? There seems to be no easy answer. In important ways, selling to foundations is the same as selling to anyone else. First you have to know your customer. Many foundations, unlike health care delivery programs, have spent a lot of time formulating a mission, goals, objectives, and strategies. One useful purpose this serves is to give foundation officials good reasons to say "no," even to what they say are wonderful proposals.

Second, you have to build yourself a track record. Or rather your organization has to demonstrate accomplishment in the area for which you are requesting the funds. This is sort of like going to the bank for a loan; the bankers will only loan you the money if you don't really need it when you have ample collateral. How is your organization going to establish a track record in an area for which it lacks the capital to get started without some kind of financial help?

Third, it helps to have an "in" at the foundation, someone who knows you personally, trusts you, believes in what your organization is trying to accomplish and would like to help you, certainly not if your proposal isn't worth funding, but yes, if you have written a good proposal that fits within the foundation's guidelines. Then it helps if you are allowed to submit a draft, get feedback, and revise your proposal accordingly. Of course there are so many good causes in health care that even the substantial foundation largesse that is around doesn't go very far, and often foundations like to give large chunks to organizations "those who already have," rather than to those who are "trying to get."

Supposing that you are fortunate enough to obtain a large grant, my advice is as follows: Always consider what you have to show to get a followup grant, and organize your work accordingly. Next, what do you have to do to satisfy your project officer so that there will not be "any trouble," and so that your project officer can "look good?" Isn't this easy? Just do whatever it was that you said you were going to do in the grant, however you said you were going to do it. But what if circumstances change? And they always do. Then, as early on as possible, go and talk to your project officer, face to face, explain the changing circumstances, tell them your suggested response, and ask them for their advice and do what they suggest to do. What if you don't want to do as they suggest? Then, give back the money; this is the only honorable thing to do. Or beg their forgiveness. What many grantees do instead is to delay and hope that foundation officials will change their minds or forget about whatever it was that they wanted you to do, in the face of other priorities. Maybe something will turn up. My experience tells me that this doesn't work. The key as always is a good fit between the project coordinator's vision of the grant and the project officer's vision. Trust on both sides, and a sound proposal with regular reporting generally results in a win/win outcome, but these are not always normal conditions.

Working with Foundations: A Checklist

Yes	No	
_____	_____	Do you know the priorities of local and national foundations regarding the programs you wish to seek funding for?
_____	_____	Has your organization established any kind of a "track record" in these programs or related program areas?
_____	_____	Does your organization regularly network with foundation officials (either through a fund-raiser and/or by attending meetings at which foundation officials explain their priorities)?

_____ _____   After the grant is awarded, does your organization do what you said would be done, or else, do you meet with the project officer early on to suggest possible changes?

_____ _____   Do you always have a handful of ideas, regarding programs your organization would like to start or expand, if foundation support were available?

_____ _____   Do you know how to write a good grant that fully complies with foundation guidelines?

_____ _____   Do you understand that in dealings with your project officer, she is always "right," if you want to receive further grants from that foundation?

Practical Exercise

Go to the library (or use the Internet) to find out the names of 5–10 foundations, including two or three local foundations and read up on their missions, goals, and objectives. From the list, write to two or three of these foundations and ask for a meeting to learn more about their funding priorities, assuming there is already a good fit between projects they fund and projects for which you are seeking funding. Send them in advance information about your organization and yourself, and about some of the programs for which you may be seeking support, and which cannot be undertaken without such support. Be ready to show evidence of efforts at collaboration with other providers or of other funding which you have obtained. Go to the meeting with three of four projects in mind, ask whether the foundation might be interested, and seek their advice regarding either funding from them or from another foundation.

8

Governing Nonprofits

I joined the governing board of the Lutheran Medical Center in 1983, and as of 1998, still serve. I have also served on the governing boards of the following organizations: First Professional Bank (a for-profit bank, listed on the American Stock Exchange which serves mainly physicians), the Metropolitan Health Plan, a Detroit HMO, the Association of University Programs of Health Administration, and the Augustana Nursing Home, all stints lasting three years or less, in addition to consulting to several nonprofit organizations on improving board effectiveness. I also constructed the Board of Governors' examination on governance for Fellowship in the American College of Healthcare Executives. I was also a member for several years of a study group of academics, across sectors, interested in nonprofit governance and funded by the Lilly Endowment.

With Tom Holland and Roger Ritvo, I have written a book, *Improving Board Effectiveness,* published in 1997, and several chapters in other books and articles on nonprofit governance, including "Improving Hospital Board Effectiveness: An Update," published in *Frontiers of Health Services Management* in 1990, winner of the Conley Award, from the American College of Healthcare Executives, as the outstanding health care article of the year.

What the Literature Says About Nonprofit Governance

What I have learned from the literature is as follows: There is no theory or accepted model of how boards affect organizational performance or regarding mechanisms of accountability to stakeholders. There is some agreement on board functions. Different organizational sponsors surely have different organizational objectives. For boards to add value, they must have their own work to do.

Sofaer and others (1994) have argued that relative to how hospital trustees actually behave or what they actually do, the literature does not include "a theory or model of how the board can directly affect the performance of hospitals; an articulation of the most appropriate size or composition of a governing body for a particular institution; or, a relation of specific behaviors of governing bodies to performance measures of hospitals."

A central governance issue for nonprofits is how to enhance accountability when nonprofit boards do not specify measurable objectives for themselves or for organizational performance, when board members are not selected based primarily on required skills and experience, that is, to guide strategic planning and evaluate top management; and, when chief executives do not want strong boards.

Mintzberg (1983) has posited that boards have these functions: to select and evaluate the chief executive, to exercise direct control during periods of crisis, to review managerial decisions and performance, to coopt (persuade) external influencers, to establish contacts and raise funds, to enhance the organization's reputation, and to give advice. He suggests that, except under extraordinary circumstances, boards do not make strategic decisions.

Different sponsors of nonprofits, such as hospitals, have different objectives. For example, physicians and investors may seek profit; cooperatives and unions, services, and jobs for their members; government, votes; churches, believers; employers, lower health care costs; and philanthropists, prestige.

According to Drucker (1989), "in the effective nonprofit, every board committee, every board member, accepts a work program with specific achievement goals. So does the chief executive officer, with regular appraisal against pre-established performance goals; and, with resignations, if performance consistently falls below goals and expectations." Of course, a lot more has been written about hospital and health system governance of nonprofits, but this is not our concern here, other than to say there is not much science on which to base practical experience.

My Board Experience at Lutheran Medical Center

In 1980, I edited a special issue of *New York Affairs*, "Health in New York: A Progress Report," which contained interviews by B. Jacobs (1981) of managers in four local innovative health care organizations—one was Lutheran Medical Center. At about that time, I had a conversation with the CEO, George Adams, to see if I could interest him in working more closely with the health program of the Wagner School (of which I was then director). Lutheran ran a large neighborhood health center, similar to Gouverneur's, in southwest Brooklyn, funded by Lyndon Johnson's Office of Economic Opportunity.

New York Affairs described Adams as "LMC's smooth-and-dapper, silver-haired president." He had gotten into health care management in part to rectify the terrible care he and his family received at a municipal hospital when he was a poor kid in one of the outer boroughs. As a youth, while applying for a driver's license, he had been kept outside in the cold waiting by government officials, while others were being served inside; then, the state officials closed the doors at 4:30 PM, saying they were closed for the day (official hours ended at 5:00 PM).

Adams' point was that the state officials thought that "this was their facility," but "we the public were paying their salaries and this was really *our* facility. No one in business would have run a service operation the way they were running this operation." Adams added that the trouble with hospital administrators was that they thought they were running their places to serve the doctors or not to lose money, but what they should have been doing was serving the folks who lived in the community and used (or should have been using) the hospital, which was just another building. Serving the neighbors was the basis for all the decisions Adams made at Lutheran, from teaching local immigrants how to speak English so that they could find jobs, to constructing housing for older people because that was what the people in the neighborhood needed most. (Yes, most people viewed his job as running the hospital facility).

Adams told me about the importance of the way things looked for the people who were running the hospital. For instance, he wouldn't stand for one of his managers buying meat from a hospital purveyor at a steep discount—it wouldn't look right. Now retired, Adams was a tremendously successful nonprofit manager, who stayed at Lutheran for more than 30 years, retiring while he was still ahead. Adams led Lutheran to national recognition for community service (Lutheran was also one of the 49 hospital community benefit grantees in our Kellogg demonstration program). He initiated new facilities and programs and developed a loyal and effective top management team. Adams was fortunate to work with Howard Smith, Lutheran's board chair throughout his tenure. A successful businessman, Smith supported Adams consistently and predictably, and was responsible in some considerable part for Adams' and the hospital's success.

When I met George Adams for the first time, I told him of my interest in hospital boards as an academic field of study, and I asked whether there was a chance that I could work with him as a member of Lutheran's board. Adams said something might be worked out. He said that I could attend board meetings, but that unless I was of the Lutheran faith, there wasn't much chance of my serving, since half the board members had to be Lutheran, as this was a church-sponsored hospital. Luckily for me, I had converted to Lutheranism in Detroit after my marriage to Chris, and I became a board member at Lutheran in 1983.

Adams' view and my own of hospital boards couldn't be more different. He preferred a rubber stamp board with a powerful supporting chair with whom he worked as a team. He feared a micro-managing board, and the board chair shared his view. In this way, Adams' power, as CEO, was then maximized to do good for the community. And Lutheran Medical Center has done a great deal of good for its community all these years.

During my tenure as a board member, Lutheran has not specified measurable objectives, nor formally articulated organizational goals shared with stakeholders. There was no formal evaluation of the CEO until after Adams' retirement. Until recently, no strategic plan existed, and the one that exists now was mainly developed by consultants. Recently also, as a result of guidelines from the Joint Commission on the Accreditation of Health Care Organizations, Lutheran has formulated some general goals and adopted a mission statement. A committee of the board now formally evaluates and sets compensation for the CEO. Although board members were given by Adams' successor, a copy of my book, "On Improving Board Effectiveness," none of the board members has ever spoken with me or discussed with me how, if at all, the book applies to Lutheran, where the board falls short, and what, if anything, the board should do about it.

My Experience Consulting to Boards

My three main consultancy assignments to boards have been to a university, a specialty college of physicians, and to a small health system. My approach, in each case, was to interview several trustees to understand how they viewed present circumstances, and to learn what they saw as current problems and issues. Subsequently, I shared this information with a steering committee of the board and with the CEO, in order to plan a board retreat. At the retreat, the full board would be provided with the information with which they had previously supplied individually. The steering committee would decide in advance what directions they wanted actions to be recommended. By the close of the retreat, the trustees would hopefully reach agreement on new directions and the strategy for implementation, agreeing on responsibility specified and time lines for implementation. Of course, events did not always work out according to plan.

The University

The president of a university invited me to serve as a consultant to the board of trustees. The president wanted a better functioning board that would add more value. I made a number of suggestions. For example, there were not enough board members who were passionate about the university and who brought relevant skills, experience, or representation to the table. A step in the right direction had been made in terms of fixed terms of office, but the board was very large. I suggested contrasting the present with the desired board composition in terms of skills, resource generating potential, and other attributes, to include geographical distribution and diversity. I suggested that the nominating committee be more vigorous in ending service for some board members at one term, and that the chair be more active in telling board members what was expected and in encouraging nonperformers to step up to what was expected of them or more usually to withdraw. I pointed out the duplication in agendas between the executive committee and the board meetings. Board meetings were repetitious for members of the executive committee, while board members not on the executive committee felt that they had less status as they only discussed policy after this had been digested by the executive committee.

I raised questions about whether the board's job was solely to recruit, support, and evaluate the president. The board could choose to add value in other ways, for example, by helping to shape the strategic future of the university. Another issue of responsibility was the board's willingness to be accountable for raising money either directly by giving or by assisting in university fundraising, with a target set for the board to attain. I suggested adequate job descriptions for board members, orientation, and continuing education for trustees, and that the board have objectives for itself which are measurable and set in advance every year.

I suggested that the board committee structure be reexamined with a view to eliminating committees and reducing membership where committees were too large. The following committees might be eliminated or combined with others: honorary degrees, investment, physical facilities, university health services, and student affairs. Development could be spun off as the primary activity of a separate board and not be part of the board of trustees as such. Consideration of new committees or of functions which should be important mandates of existing committees were the following: strategic planning, quality assurance or oversight, and relationships with a religious sponsoring community. I suggested that committees would be more effective if chairs established measurable objectives annually, together with the board chair and president, and reported on quarterly progress in goal attainment throughout the year.

There was a general preference among board members whom I interviewed that the board spend more of its collective effort on strategic rather than tactical or current issues. I suggested this concern could be addressed by increased staff support to the board and by altering the timing and content of board agendas. For example, time could be spent analyzing innovative universities and the implications for the university of their new approaches to teaching and research. I suggested that consideration be given to developing a set of critical indicators comparing the university's performance to comparable universities and with its own historical performance. Other issues I identified were the ineffective leadership of the board chair, inadequate feedback given to board constituencies, and ineffective processes by which the board did its work.

The board, however, failed, over the short run, to implement my suggestions. Although the president was favorably impressed with my work, he accepted another position, and improving governance had been his project. The planned retreat never took place, and I was never contacted by his successor.

The College of Physicians

My experience at the college of physicians was more successful—the board retreat eventually took place. I was hired by a single-term, nonsalaried president and supported by the salaried chief administrative officer. I made the following recommendations to the board.

The board should focus on critical indicators of college performance relating to mission, goals and objectives, membership satisfaction and participation, revenues and expenses and uses of capital, appropriate use of staff, influencing and adapting to governmental policy and trends, and self-evaluation. Board meetings should have shorter agendas and better developed agenda books, new board members be formally oriented, the board evaluate its own performance, with regular reporting on progress in implementing strategic plans, more delegation of current board work to college councils and committees, and review of the frequency and length of board meetings.

The board should arrange for better matching of college financial and manpower resources with strategic priorities, more appropriate division of work between the college and subspecialist societies, other specialty organizations and nonspecialty medical organizations, such as the American Medical Association. Councils of the college should develop their own priorities and work plans and present them to the College Board of Directors for review.

Again, many of my suggestions were not implemented over the short run. Possible explanations are that the college, perhaps, had more pressing priorities, that this was the president's, and not the board's project, or that by the time I had been hired, worked with the steering committee, facilitated the retreat, disseminated the findings, the president's term was over, and so, the project was over.

The Health System

The base hospital for the health system, which I consulted for, was founded in 1867 and had 475 licensed beds and 120 extended care beds, and provided general acute care and specialty services to residents of three urban and suburban counties. The health system is located in a suburban community, near New York City. At the outset of the project, the health system comprised six corporations, including a parent that elected trustees of the other five. There were 26 board members of the parent board, half of whom were aged 65 and over and who averaged almost 30 years of service. Standing committees of the board included executive, finance/audit, nominating, joint conference, buildings and grounds, pastoral care, and quality assurance.

Over a 3-year period, under a Lilly Foundation grant, along with Roger Ritvo and Tom Holland, I worked closely with the board. We focused on a number of areas: assessing board strengths and limitations, conducting a variety of training and coaching procedures, examining trustees' learning styles and approaches to their tasks, strengthening their practical mastery of board skills and their application to issues before the board, monitoring the effects of these efforts upon board performance, and documenting the patterns and consequences of changes in board behavior.

After identifying, screening, selecting, and confirming the health system as one of six nonprofits that would participate in the project, we oriented the board and conducted initial assessment of current performance in each of six competency areas. For example, one competency area was the political dimension—the board accepts as one of its primary responsibilities the need to develop and maintain healthy relationships among key constituencies. We used a board self-assessment questionnaire that invited trustee observations about board activities in these areas. We also conducted diagnostic interviews with selected leaders of the board, examining board performance in the six areas, and identifying aspects of board performance that were strong or weak. From the findings of these steps, we prepared profiles of board performance highlighting aspects that needed attention in subsequent steps of board development.

At the initial retreat with the board, we presented a summary of the findings of the interviews and questionnaires from their trustees. Participants discussed their concerns about board performance and then set priorities for our work together during the project time period. Among the techniques we used to develop their plans were reflections on responses to the contents of the assessment report, case studies, and small group work sessions on formulating priorities. The retreat concluded with group exercises that led to selection of a few priority issues for attention and work over the coming months.

Over the following months, we provided facilitation, coaching, and consultation to the boards, while the members worked on strengthening their competencies in addressing the board's substantive concerns. We observed at board and committee meetings, provided feedback and suggestions on issues that arose in work on agenda items, and met with board leaders and ad hoc committees to monitor progress and to develop plans for further steps to improve board performance.

The health system board implemented the following steps subsequent to its first retreat: reduced the number of system boards from six to four; established term limits for board members; selected new chairs for the parent board and for the hospital (the previous hospital board chair had served for 17 years); reduced the size of the hospital board from 26 to 17 (phased in over a 3-year period); approved a roster of educational programs for presentation at the quarterly board meetings; implemented a consent agenda for board meetings (minor items grouped for voting without extensive discussion); reorganized the hospital's board committee structure as executive/finance, board development, quality improvement, community benefit, and strategic planning; expanded membership on board committees to allow service by persons not on the board; diversified the board by adding more women; and developed a trustee orientation manual for new members. Areas that the board identified for future attention included setting measurable objectives for the board (against which board performance could be evaluated); developing strategies to improve board-staff relationships; formulating criteria and steps for measuring quality of performance; assessing consumer needs and determining scope of services; responding appropriately to environmental pressures, such as government regulation; and, assuring hospital competitiveness by keeping pace with technology.

These steps were recommended or considered as leading toward improved board performance. Performance was self-defined by the board and emphasized enhancing of board competencies or the board's adding value to attaining objectives in the strategic plan and preparing for adaptation to future competitive pressures. For example, reducing the number of boards from six to four enhanced the hospital board's strategic capability through requiring a number of key trustees to attend fewer total board meetings and to focus on fewer institutions.

Many of our suggestions were implemented by the health system board. What happened over the short term, subsequently, was that a significant group of attending physicians at the base hospital allied themselves with a larger neighboring health care system. The CEO, who had hired us as consultants, was persuaded to leave, as the trustees gave over operating control to the larger health system. And so, although the operation was a success, in a sense, the patient died. The board still exists, but it has become advisory to the board of the larger health system.

Unifying Ideas

To my mind, none of these three boards saw that there was anything seriously wrong. For them reforming ineffective governance, was not a high priority. The president of the university would, I believe, have carried out reforms if he had stayed on the job, the president of the college lacked the power and authority to implement the changes, and the CEO of the health system lacked support from the board chair, board members with necessary skills and experience, or other medical staff leaders with vision who could have enabled the CEO and the health system to weather the political storm.

Working with Scholars on Nonprofit Governance

In the early 1990s, for about 5 years, the Lilly Endowment funded a study group of which I was a part. Formed by Professor Richard Chait, then at the University of Maryland, funded by the Lilly Endowment, the group studied nonprofit governance. Membership in the group has been one of my most pleasurable experiences in academia.

There were about 12 members in the group, most of whom were academics. I was nominated, as a health sector expert, by the director of the American Hospital Association's Research and Educational Trust. Other nonprofit sectors represented included religion, social welfare, art, and education. We met every three or four months in a different hideaway usually in a rural setting. We'd bring in a famous visitor to talk about his work, such as Professors Amitai Etzioni or Richard McClelland. The next day we'd talk about our own work, having sent to each other in the interim, articles and book suggestions. The group was highly collegial.

The two members with the strongest points of view were Dick Chait and Tom Holland, who were collaborators with Barbara Taylor, also a member of our group, on another Lilly Endowment project. They published together two excellent books, *The Effective Board of Trustees* (1991) and *Improving the Performance of Governing Boards* (1996). Dick Chait shared with the group his frustration at the limited accomplishments of most boards (a frustration shared by many of our members). Tom Holland, an excellent methodologist, was concerned with measuring, in a valid and reliable way, the actual behavior of boards, and the impact of consultant interventions on board behavior.

In their first book, Chait, Holland, and Taylor tried to answer the following questions: (1) What characteristics define and describe effective boards of trustees of independent colleges? (2) Do the behaviors of effective and ineffective boards differ systematically? (3) What is the relationship, if any, between board effectiveness and institutional performance? Their findings were: there are specific characteristics that distinguish strong boards from weak boards; there is a positive and systematic association between the board's performance, as measured against these competencies, and the college's performance, as measured against some conventional financial indicators; and, self-assessments by board of trustees are of questionable validity as accurate and objective measures of actual board performance and competence.

In their second book, the authors tackled a new question "Can boards of trustees learn to improve, to become more competent?" They screened and selected six colleges based upon three major factors: (1) the motivations of the president and the board chair to participate; (2) excluding any college in the throes of organizational crisis; and, (3) the value, for research purposes of ensuring some diversity among institutions. For 36 months, they worked with each board to improve performance. (The study was replicated by Holland, Ritvo, and myself, resulting in the publication "Improving Board Effectiveness: Practical Lessons for Nonprofit Health Care Institutions," 1997.) After 10 years of research and dozens of engagements as consultants to nonprofit boards, Chait, Holland, and Taylor reached a rather stark conclusion that *effective governance by a board of trustees is a relatively rare and unnatural act.* This conclusion is verified by my own experience. They divided board competencies into two groups. The contextual, educational, analytic, and strategic dimensions are essentially cognitive skills; all four involve the board's capacity to learn, analyze, decide, and act. The interpersonal and political dimensions concern affective or relational skills, oriented more toward process than substance. But the authors concluded that even with these competencies, boards have only marginal utility unless these assets engender decisions and actions that add value to the institution. These decisions and actions can be facilitated by the board's helping senior management determine what matters most; creating opportunities for the president to think aloud; encouraging experimentation; monitoring progress and performance and modeling the desired behaviors.

I have had some difficulty squaring the authors' emphasis with my own experience. Simply put, I have found that most boards don't see it as in their interest to change toward becoming more effective. Board members don't want to admit as a group that they don't function very well. Most CEOs won't admit that they would just as soon prefer the board to be powerless. So the basic question becomes, in my view, how do you get the board *ready* to do what they should, rather than what should be changed and how should we change it. Chait, Holland, and Taylor write that the first step toward board development is to create a sense of anxiety that attracts the trustees' attention, that is within an atmosphere of psychological safety that reassures the participants that change is both desirable and feasible. Frankly, I think a whole book could and should be written on how to get the board ready for change. The easy answer is to say what we need is leaders with vision who understand the problem and whom the board trust. This answer, it seems to me, is too easy. My experience tells me that effective leaders are likely to have other more important priorities and that board members who trust such leaders in general don't trust them on this one; besides there is a risk to the leader in messing with the board that his own job tenure or autonomy will be threatened.

I see the key to effective leadership as vision from the board chair. The problem here is that a new board chair is likely to have other priorities; an old board chair is likely to be too defensive about his own behavior. So if improved governance is to have higher priority, perhaps this must be demanded by powerful external stakeholders of the organization who see and demand better board performance because better boards have achieved results that they want to see achieved. Evidence of such performance is today largely lacking for the nonprofits, I know, evidence from Chait, Holland, and Taylor to the contrary. They did show that financial performance of colleges where the boards scored better on the study competencies was better, but to what extent is this going to convince any board to make significant changes, colleges even, not to mention other nonprofits? What Chait, Holland, and Taylor recommended, as a process, is fairly expensive certainly in terms of the time of trustees and managers. Well-managed retreats are an important component of improving board effectiveness. Many nonprofit board members cannot stomach the idea of going away on a retreat where they might find fault with themselves, or for any purpose.

An Agenda for Governance at Lutheran Medical Center

Lutheran Medical Center is a large community hospital (over 500 beds). The parent corporation owns as well a medium-sized HMO (30,000 members), a medium-sized nursing home (250 beds), numerous housing projects for the elderly, a large neighborhood health center, and other smaller units, all of which, as of 1998, are currently breaking even or operating at a modest surplus. LMC is affiliated for medical education with SUNY Downstate, and for health services with the Mount Sinai-NYU Health System. The board has made the decision to pursue an affiliation-toward merger with Maimonides Medical Center, a larger medical center, also in Brooklyn, on a 50/50 board member basis, with the Lutheran board chair, Howard Smith, to be chair of L/M and Stan Brezenoff, the Maimonides CEO, to be the L/M CEO.

The current Lutheran board has 25 members. 12 of these plus three physicians are slotted to be board members of the new L/M corporation. Currently, half the LMC board is Lutheran and half the board is female. The great majority of the LMC board members live in Brooklyn, and the board is appointed by the Evangelical Lutheran Church, headquartered in Chicago, IL, which owns the medical center. There are three pastors on the LMC board, and only a few board members have business experience. Other than the board chair, there are no CEOs of even medium-sized companies or health care organizations. The board meets monthly, alternating board meetings with strategy and finance committee meetings to which all board members are invited. The board has few committees, such as nominating, finance, and joint conference (board-physician), and most of the board work is carried out by the board chair and the CEO, with decisions being ratified at board meetings. Board meetings generally run three hours, and, after a prayer, are consumed by reports by the chair, the CEO, the chief financial officer, the president of the medical staff, the vice president for quality of care, and the vice president for community relations, with perhaps 15 minutes to a half hour consumed by discussion of a special project such as new construction, or malpractice experience. Board meetings are collegial and friendly, and decisions are made by consensus.

LMC has been successful, starting with little or nothing, so to speak, other than our mission, and has grown substantially, primarily through the leadership and vision of our chair and CEO for over 20 years and due to generous governmental funding. This funding has been primarily from Medicare and Medicaid, but also through federal funding of our neighborhood health center, and New York state funding for the uninsured and for medical education. LMC still has problems with its board, however. From where I sit, the basic problem is that the board does not get the information that it requires to carry out its functions of guiding long-range planning and evaluating top management. We do not set explicit goals each year nor do we monitor annual progress in goal attainment for customer satisfaction, cost, volume, quality, and employee satisfaction. Some administrators, however, are working on a preliminary version of a new governance information system, as of 1998, per my request made a year previous.

I would focus reform efforts primarily on restructuring two board committees: (1) Nominations and Board Development; and, (2) Management and Organizational Evaluation. The functions of the former committee would be, first, evaluation of the skills and experience of the current board in relation to what would be required to carry out its assumed functions of guiding long-range planning and evaluation of top management. Some types who are missing from the LMC board are CEOs from other businesses and from noncompeting health care organizations, and individuals with expertise in health care of populations, strategic planning, and information systems. Second, the committee should plan a vigorous program of board education and self evaluation. This should include learning from best practice nonprofit boards and best practice organizations in areas such as quality improvement and employee satisfaction. In terms of getting value from board members, the board chair should proactively manage the board, reviewing in advance with each board member how each can contribute, and seeing whether the board member is willing and able to do so. If the board member does not contribute as agreed, with no satisfactory reasons for noncompliance, the board member should be expected to resign gracefully.

The functions of the management and organizational evaluation committee would be to evaluate top management and fix compensation, and to evaluate organizational performance. Regarding the latter, the committee should obtain board agreement on some number of core and urgent benchmarks (say 10 of each), monitor quarterly current organizational performance relative to the indicators and targets for each indicator, and decide, at least annually whether the indicators and targets should be changed. Core benchmarks provide long-term measures of organizational performance, while urgent benchmarks deal with short-term objectives. For example, long-term measures might pertain to financial health and development of top management, while shorter term objectives might focus on financial operating performance and infection rates.

The committee should set short-term and longer term objectives, in evaluating management performance, which obviously bear a close relationship to the organizational performance objectives. There may well be areas over which top management has greater control or can make a greater contribution to attainment of objectives. The committee would have to decide which managers are to be included in top management, and should monitor learning plans as well as compensation for these individuals. Performance bonuses should be included as part of compensation, with pay levels set low enough in the case that management is currently overcompensated for current poor performance. With both committees, the committee chair should set out in advance (with board chair approval) committee performance objectives for the year and strategies to achieve the objectives, reporting back to the board each quarter on progress or lack of the same.

Third, I would like to improve the process of board meetings. All current oral reporting should be written up, distributed to the board in advance, and approved by consent at the beginning of the meeting. If any board member objects to anything in any of the reports or wants further information, he or she should have tried first to get satisfaction prior to the meetings; and if still not satisfied, by all means the item in question should be removed from the consent agenda, and discussed by the board, as currently. Then, most of the board meeting, it seems to me, can be devoted to discussing progress in implementing the organization's current approved strategic plan, with reasons given for any lack of progress and/or suggestions made for changes in the plan. Most of the rest of each meeting can then be devoted to board development, with readings distributed in advance about a topic or question.

Reflection: Governing Nonprofits

Why care about the way nonprofit organizations are governed? If these organizations are governed well, they prosper. If they fail, then perhaps they should fail. No organization should go on forever. And what do these boards do anyway, other than rubber stamp the decisions of the CEO? What should they do? Consider these examples:

1. Lou White, CEO, would like to get more fund-raising done by his board. Some board members do not give, and many give little. When asked, a common response is that board members give what they can. The board chair is unwilling to tell board members either to make or arrange for substantial gifts or to resign from the board.

2. When Tony Kovner, board member, asks the CEO whether the board could get information critical to the functions the board was expected to serve, such as information about market share, provider attitudes toward the organization, quality improvement relative to best practices at comparable institutions, he is told that *this was a wonderful idea but that the CEO had more important things to do.*

3. Clark Williams, board chair, would like to get rid of a lot of the "dead wood" on his board, but he also realizes that asking board members to resign would hurt a lot of loyal people's feelings, recruiting new board members is difficult, and present board members can be counted upon in a crisis to "do the right thing."

The question then is for the CEO: "How do I get the most out of my board?" A follow-up question for the CEO is surely, "Well, what do you want to get out of your board?" Is the important thing for board members to raise money, or to provide work, wisdom, or "wallop" (i.e., political leverage)? Let us assume that the board primarily adds value through its contribution to organizational long-range investment, in the widest sense, including human capital and organizational relationships and collaborations, and by monitoring organizational and CEO performance relative to mission. What is the CEO to do, when the current board does none of the above very well, and when the board chair does not see that "there is a problem"?

The CEO can do nothing, and try to show the implications of doing nothing. Or he can respond, as many CEOs do, to "hire a consultant," or similarly "to hire a consultant and conduct a board retreat." My response as a consultant is to describe for the board chair, for a small ad hoc board committee, and then for the whole board: (1) What are the facts of the situation: what does the board do, and how does the board conduct its business?; (2) What problems or concerns flow from the current situation?; and, (3) How can the board behave differently based on best practices at comparable organizations? Recommendations must be "realistic" in light of the resources of the organization, and "aligned" relative to the interests of the powers that be, as board members must see that any changes recommended are going to be in their interest (as related to organizational mission), which is usually "the rub."

To get the board "ready" to consider change, there must be frequent and patient CEO communication with the board chair, indicating current performance and how this can be improved based on best practices. The board governance information system must be redesigned so that board members get information and can raise questions about productivity, growth, quality, and customer satisfaction. The board nominating committee should include board development as a function, and recruit a bloc of new board members who understand the business and bring relevant skills, experience, and values to the table. An effective board does not micromanage, but rather adds value by doing its own work, a large part of which is effective monitoring of relationships with current and future stakeholders.

The job of the board chair is to manage the board. Key to doing this well is meeting individually with each board member and negotiating expected contribution, and then after 12 months, reviewing whether expectations have been achieved or the reasons for nonperformance. It should be understood that when board members do not do what they have agreed to do, assuming no renegotiation which can be perfectly justifiable for a variety of reasons, then resignation is expected, and if not given, requested.

Improving Board Performance: A Checklist

Yes	No	
_____	_____	Does the CEO know how well the board is performing?
_____	_____	Does the board have its own work to do?
_____	_____	Does the board get the information that it needs to carry out its expected functions?
_____	_____	Is there clarity as to how the board is expected to add value?

_____ _____ Does the board evaluate itself relative to measurable objectives relative to what it and the CEO expect the board to do?

_____ _____ Are expectations of the board relative to fundraising made clear to prospective board members?

_____ _____ Does the board chair see a key part of his job as "managing the board?"

_____ _____ Do board members understand what is expected of them, and are they evaluated as to whether they annually attain such expectations?

Practical Exercise

To get a better handle on how well your board of directors is doing, examine in detail board minutes (and observe a board meeting). What information, if any, is distributed in advance of the meeting? What information is routinely given to board members regarding organizational performance? What questions do board members ask routinely about such performance? How much of the meeting is taken up with reports from the board chair, the CEO, and other managers? How much of each meeting is spent reviewing progress regarding implementation of the plan for organizational performance this year? How much of the meeting is spent educating board members regarding various aspects of organizational performance? How many questions do board members ask, and what percent of the meeting is devoted to discussion of issues raised by or reacted to by members of the board?

9

Managing in Academia: A Reprise

After leaving Anytown Hospital in 1979, I was not comfortable with the idea of being an assistant director or an associate director in a hospital. I called all my friends, and as luck would have it, there was a position available as faculty member and director of the graduate program in Health Policy, Planning and Administration at NYU's Graduate School of Administration.

I liked the idea of returning home to New York City. I had been away nine years. Dean Dick Netzer explained that the school needed a director of the health program. It was in a bad state, although the program was filled with part-time health students. Several faculty had resigned, and the program lacked accreditation. Netzer explained the situation positively—it was an opportunity to make several hires and to develop the program. Its main competitors at Columbia and Baruch universities were at a similar level. The school would consider me for tenure after one year and hire me at the level of full professor. Without spending a lot of time pursuing other options, I accepted the position.

GPA (Now, the Wagner School)

The Graduate School of Public Administration (GPA), founded in 1938, is one of 14 schools at New York University, the largest private university in the United States. NYU has over 40,000 students and 2,500 faculty. NYU, at that time, owned a large university hospital as well (since merged with Mount Sinai). In 1979, GPA was one of the smallest schools at

NYU with less than 1% of budget (under $6 million), with about 700 students, most of whom were part-time, and 25–30 full-time faculty. (Eight of these faculty remain at the school 20 years later).

Netzer resigned as dean in 1981, but stayed on as a faculty member. In his valedictory report on the state of the school, he defined the school's educational and research interests as extending to all levels of government, the nonprofit sector (especially in health) and private-sector activities and organizations heavily involved with government and public policy. The geographic focus was on the New York region, serving both mid-career and pre-career students. Something he saw as uncommon in 1981, was a school of public administration, in which a majority of students were part-timers but the faculty was preponderantly full-time.

During his term as dean, the school had created a core curriculum in finance, organizational behavior, statistics, accounting, and public policy for all MPA students. In the first half of the 1970s, enrollment rose rapidly to a peak in 1972–1973, and with the health program enrollment peaking in 1975–1976. At this time, NYU was going through a severe fiscal crisis, which kept the school from increasing faculty commensurately. GPA was overwhelmed by the number of students and was not able to improve quality, consolidate the core curriculum, and implement other curricular plans as hoped.

After 1975, the story was different. Enrollment then, as compared with 1981, was 50% higher, but the faculty, in 1981, was larger. Doctoral and health program enrollments had decreased drastically. Increased selectivity was aimed at reducing attrition. As of 1981, the public administration program had about 50% of the students, urban planning had 10 percent and the health program, 35 percent (other students being enrolled in the PhD or MS programs). Thus in 1981, as Dean Netzer concluded in his report, the quality of students was better than ever and still improving, and he also praised the faculty. This corresponds with my memory of GPA at that time, although I would emphasize that the variation was very great in quality among the faculty (and in the faculty's working together) and among student quality and performance. At least half the courses were taught by adjunct faculty who had full-time jobs outside of the university, and who were also of highly variable quality.

The school's reputation was rising, as evidenced by our being the first choice of applicants for the Mayor's Scholarship Program for city employees and the success of our students in competing for presidential management internships. And GPA was doing quite well in placing our graduates. We had some financial problems due mainly to external shocks, and the upgrading of the past five years which converted GPA from having a surplus to breaking even. One key concern was the shrinkage in the relative and absolute size of the public sector, since GPA was tuition-dependent, although Dean Netzer concluded that GPA was the best, not among the weakest schools in actual quality in the region and that the school and the university would have to work very hard to make sure that this was widely appreciated. The school's identity as a research-generating enterprise was in urban public policy research, an institute for which he was leaving the deanship to head up. Netzer called for the developing of better formal and informal collaborative arrangements with other parts of the University, such as with the business school (Netzer, 1981).

In 1981, I saw my task as getting the health program accredited. In order to do so, I needed to hire new faculty, and offer new and require new courses. For me, this was a task—I was accustomed to doing, and in contrast to my other jobs, something I knew how to do. Of course, I had to relate with the existing health care faculty, two of whom were former program directors, persons of stature and notable eccentrics. I remember when Elena Padilla interviewed me while I was being recruited, this was done in a conference room; she read her mail, looking up from time to time to interview me from behind sunglasses. When I visited Herb Klarman in his office, the floor was filled with papers piled high to the ceiling so that I had to walk through a maze of such piles to approach his desk. Aside from one faculty member, Chuck Brecher, who joined the faculty the same year that I did, none of the others remain, 18 years later.)

GPA was different from Wharton. The key faculty in my program were much older, and school was not as prestigious as Wharton, nor was the health program. My role, however, was more critical. Since Dean Netzer was a scholar rather than a health or a management person, he sought in me an administrator, someone who would get the health program on the right track. This gave me a lot of room to enact my goals.

In size, GPA was similar to a large academic department. Indeed, it would have been more efficient to run the school as a department in a larger school. This was how public administration was organized at Cornell where I received my MPA in the School of Business and Public Administration. Early in my tenure at NYU, discussions were held regarding merger of GPA with NYU's business school. But the faculty was hostile to merger, and their faculty was indifferent.

Programs within GPA did not have their own budgets. The full-time faculty teaching load was five courses over two semesters, with summers "off." This meant that faculty were paid to work nine months of the year. Program directors received one to three courses off for being program director, and I recall having to teach only two courses for my first academic year. For administration, the school had, at that time, a dean, a faculty member who was part-time associate dean, three program directors, and various administrators and support persons in areas such as finance and personnel, admissions and placement.

The faculty had a governance charter, passed in 1976 (and not amended as of 1998), but had limited responsibility for anything other than tenure and promotion decisions. The faculty personnel committee consisted of 11 elected faculty members; nine tenured, and two nontenured.

Lessons Learned As Program Director

The customary advice to faculty offered the job of program director is not to take it. Or, if you are persuaded to take the job, don't take it for long. No faculty member I know has ever been willing to say he or she would want or could like such a job. To me, however, due to my management background, the job was very appealing. I also saw this as a defined challenge that I could accomplish.

Indeed, I accomplished a great deal during my tenure as program director. First, I recruited a top-notch faculty—Steve Finkler in Accounting and Finance, Roger Kropf in Marketing and Information Systems, Victor Rodwin in Comparative Health Systems, and Michael Yedidia and Beth Weitzman in Health Policy. Second, I encouraged Jim Knickman to establish a Health Research Program, which became a great success under his leadership before he left to head up evaluation for The Robert Wood Johnson Foundation. Third, I pioneered the development of the Capstone Course at GPA where groups of five to seven students working under faculty supervision do consulting projects for service organizations in the community. In the health program we developed the capstones as an alternative to the school comprehensive examination; and the school eventually followed our lead. Fourth, I led the reconceptualization of our health curriculum to four subconcentrations with required courses. These were originally management, policy, finance, and human resources, the last of which we subsequently dropped for lack of demand. Again, the school followed our lead establishing concentrations for the PA students as well in management, policy, and finance. And, the health program received full accreditation from the national accrediting agency for seven years.

What made my effort successful was the full support of Dean Netzer and his successor, and a mandate to proceed. Circumstances were also in my favor; we had many good students and alumni, and numerous faculty vacancies. Usually, the job of program director is a routine job as deans do not want to spend scarce discretionary funds for existing programs, and other programs compete for a limited number of faculty slots. However, at GPA, the health program was fortunate as to resource allocation to be a large program in a small school.

After I had worked for ten years as program director, and Netzer had been succeeded by another dean, a new dean came in. We had personal differences over the division of functions between the dean and the program director, and I chose to focus my energies on other projects.

Health Care Management Education: Views and Opinions

I wrote an article in 1986 called "Reflections on Health Management Education," in which I lay out my views. They haven't changed much over the last 12 years. Today's professional health care manager, as always, should have a good liberal education and then a master's degree in management, best acquired after several years of work experience. I think now that managerial competencies can be measured in graduate school upon admission and at graduation, to document the value added in skills and experience of an expensive, and hopefully collaborative education. This presumes that educators know the competencies which make for effective managers. But students remain in charge of their own educations. Much of what students should be learning in graduate school does not occur in the classroom but rather from the projects and assignments that they do outside, and from the conversations students have with classmates, alumni, other preceptors, and with faculty.

In my 1986 study, several of 21 academics and practitioners, whom I interviewed regarding health care management education, said that health care managers have: (1) difficulty responding appropriately to the new environment of competition and purchaser price pressure; (2) difficulty managing changing power relations with physicians and governing boards; (3) a lack of knowledge regarding what is efficient production of health services of adequate quality; and, that (4) health care organizations make a low investment in continuing professional education and career development for managers. I believe that this still applies.

Several of those interviewed said that health care management education programs need to: (1) improve teaching methods, add to the curriculum, and learn from business; (2) form effective linkages for teaching and research between faculty and practitioners; (3) link within the university health care management and clinician faculty; and, (4) specialize, for example, some programs focusing on long-term care, or health care information systems. With regard to NYU, because of our emphasis on training part-time students, our health program is short on contact hours, with 15 courses required, mostly of two hours per week for 15 weeks, versus 19 3-hour courses at some business schools. I believe that we rely too much on the lecture method of teaching, and do no assessment (nor do our competitors) of students enrolling and graduating relative to competencies required by effective managers.

I have long favored strategic alliances between health care provider organizations and educational programs, for example, our using senior managers as adjunct professors, and the organizations using our health professors as their researchers and evaluators. My efforts have been generally met by indifference from top managers (they have more important things to do) and by hostility of faculty (who want to be free to do their own research). At NYU, the medical school leadership has long viewed our management and finance faculty as clerks, with whom no real collegial partnership was feasible.

In 1986, the interviewees suggested numerous options to improve management education. These included teaching of business innovations such as quality improvement, computerized scheduling, product line planning and marketing, and performance appraisal and incentive pay systems. They suggested that faculty participate in the design and evaluation of demonstration programs in health care organizations. Faculty and practitioners could take sabbaticals in each other's organizations. A research and evaluation unit within a health care organization could be staffed by or linked to graduate program faculty, or health care organizations could contract with the graduate faculty for research or evaluation. The school could run forums or institutes for practitioners and develop electronic information exchanges on approaches to solving problems, with list servers and chat lines managed by faculty. Our faculty has been slow to adapt in these areas, in part because university incentives do not favor such adaptation and faculty are free to do "their own thing." The reward system favors becoming an expert on a narrow subject and publishing in peer-reviewed journals, even in a professional school.

In 1986, I made the following three recommendations. Programs should consider: (1) revising curricula and exploring new methods of teaching; (2) developing closer linkages with clinician educators and health care managers; and (3) undertaking related missions of continuing professional education and multidisciplinary research and evaluation. I find these recommendations as pertinent in 1998 as they were in 1986.

As of 1998, Wagner and the health program are revising, but too slowly, curricula and the way that we teach. Today's health care managers need to understand finances and costs and to measure benefits related to such costs. They need to know how to improve quality and how to work in teams. They need to assess themselves and manage themselves in challenging and ambiguous circumstances. They need to be electronically competent. To accomplish such change, we must either expand the curriculum or take out certain material. Faculty must develop ourselves so that we can teach what is required in the way that is best for our students. Simply put, the incentives aren't yet here for faculty to see changing behavior as being in the faculty's interest. For one thing, the job market remains strong and the quality of our student body is actually improving. Tuition revenues are flat or improving.

This is not to say that individual faculty members are not swimming against the current. Faculty change and develop for several reasons. Some faculty work as highly paid consultants, teaching managers for $3,000, or more, a day. Faculty who teach marketing and information courses must keep pace with changes in the marketplace to be relevant in the classroom. Some faculty are highly interested and highly competent in electronic communications. (Roger Kropf teaches in a long-distance learning course at the University of Colorado, even as he teaches at NYU). But processes and incentives are lacking for faculty to work and learn together effectively as a group.

Our school has already worked toward developing closer linkages with clinician faculty and management practitioners. Two of our health faculty do research with clinicians at other universities. Management practitioners serve as adjunct faculty in our teaching programs and teach courses such as operations and human resources management. Our school offers 44 capstone courses with employer organizations, and practitioners sit on program advisory committees and advise on curriculum and managerial competencies. Ellen Schall, a Wagner faculty member, has developed a clinical initiative which has spurred the development of half courses in areas such as project management, conflict management, and reflecting on management. She also developed a no credit course called "immersion in management" where students shadow a senior manager for a week in a local organization. The school and program also offer students a variety of internships and residencies, some paid and some unpaid. For the student who can properly get organized and effectively network, almost an unlimited management education is available, including course work at NYU's graduate business school or at other universities.

I have been struck by the organic linkages in academic medical centers of teaching, research, and service. Each function needs separate leadership and budgets to operate properly, which often does not occur in the medical centers. But as part of a whole, all three functions are more likely to flourish when better integrated, and when the key operatives are located geographically close enough so that face-to-face contact is facilitated.

In my 1986 article, I recommended, as well, that health care management programs undertake or expand related missions of continuing professional education and multidisciplinary research and education. I am assuming that professional schools have some expertise in leading and coordinating such an effort, in assuring quality, and that the schools can develop additional resources in faculty, information, and ways of teaching, perhaps in partnership with large health care organizations or consulting firms. Organizing for nondegree education requires separate leadership and budgets within a school and staffing which will be different from degree programs. A school's competitors include consultants, trade associations, the employer institutions themselves, and the school's own faculty, who as do hospital's attending physicians, sometimes compete for revenues in a nonorganizationally affiliated capacity. Competitors of professional schools can argue, with justification, that they can do at least parts of continuing education as well if not better than the schools can, and their overhead is usually much less.

Multidisciplinary teaching and research will be carried out when school incentives favor such action. Indeed many faculty are already disposed to do such research as they recognize that multidisciplinary teams are required to carry out the work effectively. Tenure and promotion committees must favor and reward multidisciplinary work (with each author's contribution to any publication specifically identified). And deans must encourage multidisciplinary teaching by arranging workloads similar to faculty teaching solo.

One priority that I did not mention in my 1986 recommendations is the need to improve service to students. Tuition at Wagner is now over $2,000 per course, or over $16,000 per year (not including expenses for books, fees, etc.). Put another way, for a 15-week course, this is $133 per class session, more than tickets to a Broadway show.

In order to improve services to students, we must first, as many business schools do, accept health care management students only after considerable work experience, or with work experience built in as part of their Master's experience. Students with relevant experience will learn more and be better students. Second, encourage students to take charge of their own education rather than passively accepting what is offered to them. To do this students should be aided by networks of support going far beyond what a full-time faculty has to offer. Systematic contact must be managed with alumni, preceptors, adjuncts, and other researchers and practitioners. Third, students should be organized in cohorts or teams, as they are in some business schools, and encouraged and rewarded for learning together. The school should facilitate student operation of consulting and other businesses, advised by faculty, doing project work for public service organizations. Fourth, students should be assessed regarding their management competencies on admission and again before they graduate, suitably advised relative to their aims and qualifications, with documentation as to added value contributed by the school and by the students during the formal educational process.

Where is NYU's Wagner School with regard to this? As of 1998, faculty are talking about such change, but doing little. One market advantage that Wagner has, relative to business schools, is that we take students lacking work experience, and changing our policy would affect us negatively financially. Second, it takes time and money to offer faculty and students proper support services, and the school leadership does not yet see this as a funding priority. The same argument applies to operating student businesses and assessing student competencies.

Lessons Learned About Teaching

Teaching is one of the hardest things to do well and one of the easiest things to do poorly. It is difficult to do, because teaching requires knowledge of the subject matter, craft in performance, the ability to listen to students and to hear also what they are not saying, and coaching ability to help them perform better. Teaching a class is like preparing for a battle, or a team athletic game; every minute should be planned and accounted for, although of course, the teacher will have to change plans relative to variable class response. Teaching is easy to do, because often it is assumed that someone who knows how to do something can suitably teach someone else. Yet, in the field that I know best, teaching management, it is clear that skills needed to teach management are different from skills required for effective managing.

One of the travesties of doctoral education in America is that Ph.D.s aren't taught how to teach. Many do teach, often as a way of financing their doctoral studies; but usually they are never coached systematically nor are best practices of effective teachers filmed and discussed. This, of course, is due to a university system that rewards research rather than teaching.

My strengths as a teacher are, I believe, that I know the material, I involve the class, and I grade papers promptly, with helpful comments. My syllabi are well-organized and logical. My weaknesses are, perhaps, a somewhat intimidating personality or an appearance of disinterest. I've also been criticized for talking too fast.

Grading is a topic of extreme interest to students. In my classes, I do not give examinations nor do I curve grades. I give few As. Most of my grades are A- or B+. I never give a C+ since a B average is required for students to stay in good standing. I never cease to be amazed by the number of students who argue or complain about grading. During the past several years, I have given students the opportunity to redo a paper (also submitting the original) with no guarantee, of an improved grade.

In my career, I have witnessed three great teachers, Steve Finkler, Jim Knickman, and Bob Eilers. They have different strengths. Steve, a great storyteller, knows the material, communicates it well, listens to students, and is patient with them. He likes to use examples from real life. For example, he shows how the airlines use differential pricing to make health care pricing understandable. Jim's strength is his nurturing personality. He is sympathetic, caring, and protective of his students. Bob supplemented his lectures in health insurance with examples of how he had advised CEOs of the largest insurance companies, governors, or top bureaucrats about mistakes they had made or changes they should make in benefits policy or administration.

Teaching Management at Wagner

Our general management course was designed by a faculty committee. The faculty agreed to follow a common outline with regard to topics and number and weight in grading of assignments. Individual faculty were allowed to specify some different readings, assignments, and case studies. When I came to GPA, this was a course in Organizational Theory/ Behavior and most students worked for or aspired to work in government. Now this is a course in management. Most of the students work in or want to work in nonprofits, and there is more variety in the student body. The management faculty divided the course up into 15 sessions: weeks 1 and 2, course overview, the mission of, and the manager in public service organizations; weeks 3 through 5, on environment and structure; weeks 6 through 8, on managing service delivery and quality improvement; weeks 9 through 12, on managing human resources, power and politics, culture and managerial style. Students are assigned to work in teams, and the last three weeks of each semester are devoted largely to team presentations in the areas of ethics and structures of accountability, managing cultural diversity, and creating innovation and change.

The main difference between my section and those of my colleagues is that I focus the course on management of the Wagner School. If I am teaching management in a school, I want that school to be well managed. I have written a case study about the organization of our school, one of my class assignments concerns improving service to students here, and I invite one of the deans to give the session on organizational culture and management style. Regularly, I send over the best ideas of students to the deans for consideration. Last semester one of the students suggested providing each student with intensive counseling up front regarding financing their graduate education, a great idea about which the school hasn't done enough.

The health care management course has much of the same substance and structure as the course I taught 25 years ago at Wharton, and for which, with Duncan Neuhauser, we developed our two textbooks of readings and cases, now in their 5th and 6th editions, with a similar and relevant framework (Kovner & Neuhauser, 1997a, 1997b). Originally the course was divided into six topics, starting from the role of the manager, control and organizational design over which the manager has most influence, to professional integration, adaptation, and accountability, over which the manager has much less influence. Following the example of a Wagner management colleague who teaches a similar course to non-health students, I decided to shift the part of the course dealing with the manager and accountability to the core basic management course. And I allocated the material on professional integration to my three remaining topics: control, design, and adaptation. I usually use two guest lecturers to talk about continuous quality improvement or reengineering, and marketing and planning.

For assignments, students work in teams of two, and sometimes three, analyzing control, design, and adaptation in local health care organizations or units within them. They are required to specify problems and issues, and to make recommendations for change in the form of a memo to the unit manager or director. The course makes extensive use of case studies, some of which I have written, and, to make some of my points, I use several examples from my current work as a consultant, board member, or consumer. Basically, I am interested in how students can articulate their views of managerial problems and issues rather than the student's writing down what I say, or what the readings say, and then regurgitating this in class or on a paper.

I have learned that students don't like to sit in assigned seats. So I ask them to submit photographs signed on the back which I return at the end of the course. I spend enough time learning their names, and I call upon them by name. I urge students to waive the course if they already have the skills and experience. I advise students to tell me in advance if they don't want to be called upon in class; otherwise, I call upon all students regardless of whether they raise their hands. Students can improve their grades by redoing papers or by completing an extra credit assignment. I give them supplemental bibliographies, and arrange institutional introductions, as needed, to help with their team projects. The most difficulty I have is with students lacking work experience who do not understand political realities and organizational constraints.

I was asked to teach the capstone course for all management rather than only health care students and to focus on applied research rather than management solutions, as I had done previously. This capstone focuses on information which managers need to identify and respond to problems and issues. Capstone courses are challenging for students unused to relying on each other, when some members of the team lack skills, experience, or motivation, and face logistical problems related to day jobs and site locations, and client problems related to poor conceptualization of the project and lack of consistency in client wants and specifications.

I believe that the emphasis on adding value through information is a good one, rather than emphasizing recommendations about which the client has comparative advantage. I take care to choose reliable, accessible clients, seeking twice as many projects as required to give the student teams some choice. I stress with each client the importance of a doable project, the parameters of which are not significantly changed after the client has approved a team project proposal. Excellent projects are those which the client wants done, but not on an emergency basis. With the student teams, I emphasize the importance of a thorough and realistic proposal which is enthusiastically approved by the client. I stress the importance of communicating team findings in a professional way, and I rehearse each team's presentation with them before it is delivered to the client. I try to engage the Wagner school as one of the clients for the course. One semester, the student project with the school was improving alumni relations, and the team did an extensive survey of other graduate program web sites, with recommendations regarding specific features. This was a project that the school wouldn't have undertaken otherwise.

Lessons Learned Managing a Faculty

Managing a professional school faculty takes time and skill, realistic and aligned objectives and strategies, and a low and engaging managerial profile. Managing faculty is similar in many ways to managing physicians. The manager must learn what individual faculty want and how they see themselves. Faculty preferences vary among individuals and change for the same individual over time. Academics are often loners, who like to talk and see themselves as experts. To get ahead as a professor usually means becoming an expert on a narrow subject. Outside of their own discipline and program, faculty may be quite ignorant about what other faculty do. For example an urban planner who studies comparative health systems knows little about cost allocations in school finance. There is a wide range of faculty interests because they are full-time and tenured and nontenured, adjunct part-timers who are paid too little to teach a course or a few courses, and research faculty who, lacking tenure, have to live from grant revenues.

Schools such as Wagner are in multiple businesses. Our main business is masters' degree education, in public, nonprofit, and health management, policy and finance, and urban planning. Other businesses include nondegree education and research. Wagner is a small school, and being in many businesses is unlikely to achieve success in any one of them without partnering with other organizations. There are no program budgets, for example in health care, nondegree education, or research. Managing such a school is difficult and a dean can add tremendous value or cause substantial harm. Of course, many of the faculty see the school's goal as supporting them in their research and teaching.

The dean plays an important role at Wagner. Many faculty see the dean as a fund-raiser, first, last, and always, and judge the dean in terms of fund-raising performance. Even poor fund-raising performance may be forgiven if deans leave faculty alone. Occasionally deans actually do something which the faculty recognizes as for them, such as buying faculty computers or giving faculty a $1,000 allowance for travel and books. Bob Berne, the last dean before the present Dean Jo Boufford, had some outstanding decanal qualities. First, he only asked from faculty what faculty were qualified to do—namely, academic and scholarly rather than administrative work. Second, he somehow managed to focus faculty more on school objectives and strategies, that is relative to their nonschool activities, which are substantial for some faculty. He did this by focusing on a few major goals and recruiting excellent support staff which is difficult to do in universities where the pay is low, and seems only feasible when such support staff want educational benefits.

Thus, the dean's role is to decide where the school can add the most value, raise funds relative to such distinctive competence, and recruit partners to generate volume sufficient to enable low unit costs and high quality. I say this even as I have been advised in regard to dealing with a dean by other faculty that deans come and go (and I have seen five deans so far in 18 years) while the faculty stays. I have also been advised to "say yes to whatever the dean wants and then do what you want; deans never follow up and lack the wherewithal to be effective in following up."

One priority for Wagner is seeking partners, as we are too small to excel alone. Such partners include large service organizations, ranging from the Port Authority to the Mount Sinai-NYU Health System, consulting firms, and other universities. Wagner , I believe, should partner as well with other schools and programs at NYU, which include arts and science, business, law, education and nursing, social work and medicine. This latter intra-university partnering can be done only when such schools are "ready"—as I mentioned before, interschool partnership is not traditional, and requires for success strong presidential and deanly leadership and economic incentives for participating faculty.

The comparison with managing physicians in academic health centers is obvious. I see three main similarities: the inability to measure outcomes in health care or education, the multiple missions, and the lack of professional commitment to the organization. I believe that health centers are closer to the competitive pressures of the market in 1998 than are universities. No one yet approaches the college or professional school admissions officer with a deal stating "I have 25 to 30 candidates who meet your school's admission standards, and I want a 40% discount." But I believe that time is coming. The time is coming as well when schools will have fairly good data on managerial skills and experience of entering students, as HMOs acquire data on member baseline health status. Schools will then be able to measure the value of educational intervention, in coproduction with the student, over time.

An Agenda for Wagner's Health Program

As of 1998, some of the strengths of the Wagner health program are as follows: (1) we have no universally acclaimed, local competitor; (2) our health program is located in a school of public service, rather than in a school of business or public health; and, (3) Wagner has a strong and large full-time health care faculty with primary appointments in the school, and additional full-time research and clinical health care faculty. We also have a large adjunct health care faculty, who typically teach from one to two courses a year. Our current faculty areas of strength are management, to include financial management and health economics (eight faculty) and health policy, to include quantitative research (eight faculty).

Our educational program for health care managers is very good. We need to make it excellent. Some might ask, "Why become excellent?" Different faculty have different answers for this question, of course. The health program is in two other businesses as well: research and nondegree education. At present, the research activities are mainly carried out by the policy group, and the nondegree education activities by the management group.

Currently, the above activities are structured as one graduate program of health policy and management for teaching purposes. Wagner has separate research and nondegree educational programs, each of which includes a health component. My concerns and issues with the present structure are that no one on the health faculty is currently responsible for excellence in the management area (to include financial management), which is the course of study for the great majority of health program and continuing education students. There is leadership in health policy research, but not in health management research.

One recommendation I would make is to consider reorganizing the health faculty into two separate management and policy groups, with identifiable leadership and budgetary responsibility. I would strengthen the Wagner offerings in management and financial management and develop a relationship with NYU's business school (Stern) to develop specializations for our management students in the functional areas of information, marketing, human relations, and operations management. This would involve (a) Stern's encouraging Wagner students to take their classes, which may involve adding sections; and, (b) Stern's professors using health care examples in these courses. Second, Wagner management faculty should be involved in developing strategic relationships with large health care systems, such as Mount Sinai-NYU, to develop cooperative management education and research programs, using Mount Sinai-NYU managers as teaching faculty and Wagner faculty as program evaluators and management researchers.

The key constraint to implementation is that the people in power do not see my views as being of priority. To gain priority, I must demonstrate the substantial benefits to be gained by implementing my recommendations, or convince powerful persons of the logic and attractiveness of these recommendations in enhancing their own job performance. I suppose that

I would also have to put myself on the line and say that, if asked, I would be willing at a minimum to be involved in carrying out this strategy.

I would document benefits by going to the most demanding customers among our students and alumni and see what they think of these ideas. What kinds of skills do alumni employers want to see in program graduates? And how do our present graduates stack up against those from other schools? Making the changes within Wagner would be relatively easy to accomplish. I don't think the eight management faculty would object, other than to making any substantial changes in current behavior, without offsetting incentives. Under my proposal, health care management faculty would do less teaching and research, and more developing and implementing of relationships and programs with senior management in health care organizations and with Stern faculty. I would lighten the regular faculty teaching load from five to four courses for the academic year (as was implemented recently for arts and sciences faculty) to incent faculty, and appropriately support the new work responsibilities and negotiate accountability for results.

Carrying out the strategy with Stern and with Mount Sinai–NYU and other institutions requires leadership from the deans and from senior university and health system officials. It always helps if such efforts can be supported through the obtaining of outside grants and contracts. I suggest that efforts start small and build on successes. For example, Wagner could focus at first on one functional area at Stern such as information systems. This would provide opportunities for research, and encourage Stern students to take advantage of the health care management courses at Wagner. At Mount Sinai–NYU, Wagner faculty could work with senior managers on projects of mutual interest. What Wagner can offer is the opportunities for research and evaluation, for example, regarding information that Mount Sinai–NYU trustees currently and should receive. Wagner faculty can also offer management courses for Mount Sinai–NYU staff; for example, Wagner faculty could offer programs similar to the management education program for physicians that I and other colleagues offered this fall for Cornell Medical College. Mount Sinai–NYU senior managers can teach Wagner students, be clients for Wagner capstone projects, take Wagner management residents, and advise Wagner students about management careers.

The Future Beckons

So now, at age 61, I sit here at my word processor. At 59, my father was dead from cancer. My mother, at 60, had just started a new career, and worked productively for the next 25 years. Many of my peers are retired, and some have died. Because my children do not currently require financial support, and my wife Chris works—she is a tenured professor—I no longer need to work primarily for money. I see money as a useful way to allocate my time. Now, I will not engage in certain kinds of outside teaching unless I receive a substantial fee. For me, now, the primary question is how much time to spend working, and what to work on? Answering these questions is difficult.

In accordance with Russ Ackoff's advice to examine the current situation, ruthlessly, identify key problems and issues, and then develop a plan which is realistic, which is aligned with the powers that be, I present the following scenario: I currently continue, and enjoy teaching—I would prefer teaching two courses a year, rather than five courses. I work less as a consultant than I used to, which was two or three days a month. Recently, an important project for me has been to raise funds to eventually endow an annual dialogue at Wagner among practitioners and researchers to improve health care delivery. (My mother started this program with a bequest in honor of me and her parents.) Previous topics have included: "Integrated Delivery Systems: How Consultants Know What They Know," and "HMOs and Academic Health Centers: The Common Ground?" The events have been well received, with focused and articulate presenters.

Currently, I am looking for a cause or a project which will challenge my spirits and energize and focus my work, that I can conduct from my university position. Ideas include (1) better informing the public about national health insurance, starting from the premise that the 40 million Americans who lack insurance must be insured. I would like to document the state of affairs relative to the interests of the various stakeholders in health care as I have outlined before; (2) developing a health services management research center to examine issues, such as how physicians should be organized, monitored, and held accountable in complex health care organizations; (3) carrying out research on the contribution of governing boards to nonprofit organizational performance; and (4) carrying out a major management teaching and research strategic partnership with a large health care system.

Reflection: Working with Physician Managers

Managing physicians is similar to managing professors. More managers are moving away from top-down directives toward serving front-line, more highly skilled workers. Such a shift is due to managers seeing improved bottom-line results from holding front-line workers accountable, and yet empowering them within a framework of mission and prior negotiated, and frequently renegotiated, goals and strategies. Since my focus in this book is on health care management, however, I will reflect here on managing physicians rather than professors, although most of my personal experience comes from managing professors, and being managed as a professor. Consider some of the problems physician executives have in managing physicians, and other clinicians, as follows.

1. Because of her fine work in quality improvement, Dr. Sheila Winters is promoted to director of hospital quality improvement, which despite the fancy title, is a part-time managerial job. When she asks physicians to change ordering behavior often they agree and then go on as before. Or else, they disagree for unspecified reasons, such as implications for spending time or losing income, which seem to have little to do with quality-of-care issues.

2. As hospital medical director, Dr. Lalitha Sahgal has difficulty understanding what her job actually entails. Sahgal knows that she has to assure compliance with governmental regulation and help assure voluntary accreditation, work on special projects, and go to meetings with the CEO. Somehow this was not the job she had envisioned when taking it. Sahgal wonders where she got the idea that the medical director's highest priority was to drastically improve the technical and service quality of hospital care.

3. As CEO of an academic health center, Dr. Percy Swift has difficulties balancing current and long-range priorities, particularly as this impacts upon his relationships with 14 chiefs of service. Most of the chiefs were not selected based on their skills and experience as managers but rather because of their competency as researchers and teachers. And yet the chiefs are being asked to manage large departments and large budgets. Swift has suggested providing extensive and intensive management development programs for the chiefs, for which top management showed little enthusiasm.

Health care organizations underinvest in managerial development. For-profit companies, however, often spend lavishly in this area, not because they believe in the value of education, but because they believe that managerial development impacts on bottom-line results. Physicians with managerial responsibilities need the same skills and experience that any manager needs. In addition to medical production, which they presumably understand, they must value the contributions of management to the medical enterprise. Management isn't necessary just because medicine is a business; better management makes for better medicine. For example, better scheduling systems and customer feedback can facilitate patient access and trust, engendering better compliance with physician regimens and increased information for physicians concerning patient preferences and knowledge.

All physicians managers need to learn more about the craft of management, that is to say conflict and time management, financial management, budgeting and accounting, information management, quality improvement, and the financing of health care. Other important topics include professional ethics, marketing, stakeholder relations, governance, media, and community relations.

In teaching physician managers, I have not found the lecture method effective, unless the subject is primarily informational such as the history of Medicare and Medicaid or the nature of risk and capitation payment. Most of the physicians who need managerial education already have managerial jobs. Rather they must learn to analyze, in a more sophisticated way, their current political situation. How are the various customers and stakeholders being served, and what are their expectations? How do these levels of service compare with those of best practice organizations? What are the problems and issues facing physicians as managers? What are the causes of these problems and issues? How must physician behavior as managers change in ways that are realistic within the resource constraints of the organization and aligned with the political interests of those with power? What have others done in roughly similar situations? Why were the other physician managers able to succeed or why did they fail, and how does this relate to their own situations?

Physician managers need to learn from their superiors (or from other teachers) negotiating skills and teach them to their own direct reports. Over the next 12 months what results are expected? How are they achieved, and how are obstacles overcome? How will "success" be measured, and what kind of rewards can be expected if targets are attained? How can managers two levels up facilitate the negotiating process? What developmental plans will be addressed, parallel to the performance evaluation process, and how will progress be regularly monitored?

Physicians prefer to be managed by other physicians, whom they feel better share their values. They will trust physician managers more, other things being equal, when organizational change is being planned and implemented. Physicians are best influenced by data. I believe that if you give physicians relevant and focused data, the physicians will come up with their own solutions to management problems. To the extent that the physicians have front-line experience, their solutions may be better than the manager's. In any event, they are likely to generate more data and still better solutions.

Working with Physician Managers: A Checklist

Yes   No

_____ _____ Does the physician manager value management as contributing to better medicine?

_____ _____ Does the physician manager have the skills and experience necessary to carry out his responsibilities effectively?

_____ _____ Does the physician manager have a plan to obtain the skills and experience required to produce results and excel at his position?

_____ _____ Does the organization invest sufficiently in developing physician managers?

_____ _____ Do physicians managers obtain the support they need from superiors to function effectively?

_____ _____ Does top management have objectives and strategies to recruit, retain monitor, and empower physicians working for and with the organization?

_____ _____ Are physicians provided with the information they need to have sensible input to managerial recommendations for change?

_____ _____ Does top management have a validated plan to communicate with physicians and other clinicians concerning organizational goals, objectives and strategies, and regarding expectations of clinicians and from clinicians regarding organizational mission, plans, and performance?

Practical Exercise

Ask physician managers to write a paper on their career objectives and how they plan to achieve them. Discuss the following: (1) current experience in terms of managerial roles, skills, and values. Include an assessment of strengths and weaknesses; (2) desired position within 3 to 5 years. Specify the skills and experience required to obtain and excel in the desired position; (3) formulate a plan to get from #1 to #2; and, (4) determine the opportunities and constraints needed for implementation and how they will overcome constraints and take advantage of opportunities. As a second exercise for physician managers: within their current jobs, specify what are the demands or tasks that they have to do and what are the constraints or tasks that they aren't allowed to do. Between demands and constraints, what are their choices in how they spend their time and what are the most important one or two priorities, expressed in measurable terms, that they expect to achieve this year?

10

Lessons Learned in Eight Careers

Now that I have discussed management practice, teaching, and research in health care, I will focus this last chapter on career management, balancing work and life, and summarizing my views on the effective health care manager.

Career Management

In hindsight, I failed to manage my own career optimally. I believe that I could have avoided unnecessary suffering even in making the same career choices, and better equipped myself for my present responsibilities and interests. My direct experience, and my years of advising management students, however, has provided me an excellent foundation upon which I can build to advise others.

First, managers should rely on a track record that can be documented in their resume. Can you articulate how you have added value to your present employer by improving quality, increasing revenues, or decreasing costs? Update your resume, at least every year. Plan for the future what results you wish to achieve during the next 12 months and what measures you can use to portray the story you want to tell on the next revision of your resume.

Second, network, network, network. Look for opportunities to get advice from the persons who have the next job you would like to have some day. Ask them questions. What do they like about their job? What don't they like? How did they get their job? What do they have to do well in their job to succeed? At every opportunity, do favors for other people; this includes listening empathetically. Give them some reason for actively participating in your network.

Third, see where the industry is going and strategize accordingly. Why not go into a sector and into a function which is expanding rather than contracting? As of 1998, health care is moving into large firms managed as if they were smaller firms. Functional skills such as information systems and marketing are becoming more important.

Fourth, get some feedback on your "emotional intelligence," in Goleman's (1998) terms. You must learn to control your anger, and think before you speak. The first step to improving your behavior is becoming aware of your current performance, and by observing others who have developed their skills in these areas.

Fifth, find a mentor. This should be someone who will take pleasure out of helping you develop in your career. A mentor is willing to make the time to listen to you, advise you, and share his or experience in learning what you have to learn.

Finally, choose each next job carefully; try and select for goodness of fit between what the job requires and your own skills, experience, and preferences. Remember that you are more or less suited to certain jobs and situations regardless of your ability to get offers to take such positions.

Managing the Balance Between Life and Work

Life, of course, is more than work. Work played a smaller part in my parents' lives, for instance, than it has in mine. Ask yourself, what do you really want out of life? How much of what you want is determined by work? Success has different definitions for different people, too. You need to decide whether you need to support yourself alone, or with the help of a spouse, in a family with more than one job. Another version of success might be finding a job, or a series of jobs, that are not too unpleasant, putting in your hours, and getting a paycheck until it's time to retire.

Managers work in teams that achieve a level of success in the marketplace, and the manager's contribution is determined as greater or lesser in contributing to that success. No one is successful at the managerial level who is not willing to work very hard, but managers have a life apart from work. As a friend of mine says, "you can have anything but you can't have everything." So how much of the anything that you want is tied up in work? Everyone must make their own decision about this. If you don't decide, that is making a decision too.

Assuming that you want a top managerial position, work has to be a central part of your life. You've got to acquire the skills and experience to get the job and to manage effectively in the job. Managerial success depends upon the organizations you work for and the managers with whom you work. You can start working for a large organization, under the sponsorship of a powerful senior manager, and then, seek a job somewhere else, perhaps even within the same organization. Or you can work for a smaller organization, assume greater responsibility, and then seek a job somewhere else. And remember, managers always are competing with other managers in and outside your organization or unit.

I enjoy my job, largely because it is secure and I can work on projects of my choice with colleagues of my choice. Many of these projects are supported by outside funders. I enjoy teaching and developing and counseling young professional people. I enjoy serving on nonprofit governing boards. I could do a lot more than I do, but I find I have enough time for a life off the job. I love my family and spending time with them. I enjoy reading, good conversation, and food, going to movies, spectator sports, playing squash and tennis, singing, and playing the piano.

I'm glad that I have never defined myself principally in terms of the work that I do. As a result, I think I'm more fun to be around to the kinds of people I want to be spending time with. I made a decision not to be a star professor or star CEO. I chose not to pay that price. Yet I've been extremely successful—and have time to live. At 61, I can think of no greater satisfaction. I'm happy with myself.

The Effective Health Care Manager

The effective manager does what he or she is supposed to do. This can be further specified in terms of stakeholder analysis; the effective manager does what the key stakeholders expect. So what happens when key stakeholders do not agree? And what happens when the manager cannot do what the stakeholders expect (through no fault of his or her own)? To what extent can the effective manager influence stakeholder expectations so that these are appropriate?

Part of being an effective manager is figuring out what your definition of effectiveness in this job means and validating your view with key stakeholders. Typically this involves deciding what work doesn't have to be done, and what work can be done by somebody else. This assumes some vision of where the key stakeholders want the organization to be at the end of a certain period of time, as related to where they think the organization is now. There is something to be said here for George Adams' example, at Lutheran Medical Center, in telling the key stakeholders before he accepted the job what it was that he intended to do and how he intended to do it. This meant in turn that he was willing *not* to take the job if they didn't agree (of course he thought that after talking with him, they would agree.)

Even the least effective of managers with whom I have worked had character. The most effective managers are even-tempered, fair, and consistent; their management style consists of reaching agreement as to what is expected, empowering subordinates to do the job, getting them the necessary resources, and giving them the necessary support. Some of the least effective managers are exceedingly hot-tempered and inconsistent. They tell subordinates what they want done, then supervise them closely in the doing of the work. Or they talk indirectly, depending on subordinates to specify what it was that they are going to do, but refusing to be pinned down as to exactly what the managers want done or how they want it done. Subordinates are made to feel that they can never do their job as well as their boss can, and the boss's job is to teach the subordinate how to do the job right. Or, everything is fine so long as no one complains; then subordinates are confronted with the complaint and expected to rectify the matter.

I have written another book (1988) about what makes for an effective manager. Managers are confronted by various work stimuli by phone, in the mail, in conversations, and these stimuli can be grouped into episodes of management. Managers manage episodes of work, such as new construction, subordinate development, or rate negotiations. What makes for an effective manager relates to the congruence between the choices the manager makes regarding the episodes he or she manages (and how much time to spend on them) and what kind of results are produced relative to that effort, and the congruence between the episodes managed and the objectives and strategies of key stakeholders. I am assuming that the organization has articulated goals and objectives, and that evaluation is made not only regarding outcomes, which may not be within the manager's control, but according to management of processes. What matters is not only how well the manager plays his or her cards, but also what are the cards he or she is dealt.

I am now drawn to a concept of managerial effectiveness that is about a relationship between a manager and a job, rather than as being inherent in the manager himself. In other words, the same manager may be very effective in one situation and very ineffective in another. For example, I would argue that I was effective in managing the first RW Johnson Foundation demonstration program in short-term/long-term care, and unsuccessful in managing the second demonstration program in hospital-based rural health care. I had more or less the same skills and experience (actually the unsuccessful program followed the successful program, so I had more skills and experience). What was different about the two programs was a different program officer and our different relationship, and the greater specificity of the goals and strategies of the first program.

This leads me to recommend that managers spend more time evaluating the fit between their skills and experience and validating what the job requires. What I have never paid sufficient attention to in managing my own career is the importance of a good exit strategy in taking any job, figuring out in advance how to know whether the job is not working out and if that is the case what I would do next. There is always a good chance that the manager will not be the right person for the job even if the employer and the manager think that he or she is the right person. At the least, the job requirements may change, or the boss or a key subordinate or colleague may die or leave.

Reflection: On Managing Your Career

Charles Handy (1998) has estimated that on average an individual will spend 6 years working in an organization, and that for a lifetime he or she will work for six different organizations. My numbers so far approximate the average. I have worked in six different organizations over 40 years. Two of my "careers" were part time, as a consultant and a trustee. The implication is that your networks and your resume are your lifeline. Nourish them carefully. Build them on the reality of serving others and getting results in the pursuit of mission. Consider these three examples:

1. After her MBA, Sally Grant worked for a large foundation, obtained a law degree, worked in a large state as a deputy commissioner of health, had positions in government relations and health policy for two large drug companies and is now commissioner of health in a large eastern state. She is 50 years old.

2. Ann Rockport got a Masters in Hospital Administration, and has worked in the same hospital for 25 years. She has been promoted through a variety of positions and now is the CEO. Her hospital is currently merging with a neighboring and larger hospital. Ann is 48 years old.

3. After obtaining a Masters in Public Administration, Tim Bloomberg worked in a public hospital as an assistant administrator, moved to a similar position in a nonprofit hospital, then to a more senior position in an HMO, where he is currently vice president and senior network manager. Tim is 40 years old.

These people are all very successful. They too have been frustrated at work, by not having enough sufficiently challenging assignments, by not being adequately recognized, or by not being paid enough. These three managers all have, in Goleman's terms, a high emotional intelligence. This includes high self-awareness, self-regulation (the ability to think before acting), motivation to pursue goals with energy and persistence, empathy and social skills. Goleman (1998) says that such skills can be learned with practice and feedback.

But assuming the manager has high emotional intelligence, or can learn it, then what? As with everything else, it's what you can do and whom do you know. It's not enough to be competent, you have to be connected. Luck enters into it, but luck is the residue of design. The key is deciding what you want, planning how to get there, making sure that this is what you really want, and building a track record so that you can get and excel at the desired job. Another key, of course, is being satisfied with what you have. A big career is not the same as a good life. Not everyone can get to the top, and will succeed at the top. Not everyone will have a good life either, whatever that means, and no one can say whether or not he or she has a good life until we have reached the end of it. Staying healthy is certainly a big part of having a good life, and it's a necessary part of having a great career.

What continues to surprise me is the ignorance of persons in their twenties about what's out there in the way of jobs and careers and about a cold-blooded assessment of how others see you. This is why I recommend young managers network with managers five to ten years ahead of you, and ask for their advice. They should ask what the more experienced managers like or don't like about their jobs, ask them for advice about how to get such a job. Nothing succeeds like a track record of accomplishment which can be specified in terms of increased revenue, lower unit costs, improved quality of service. And, of course, this must be tied in some way to the manager's contribution, leadership or value added.

Time is the manager's most precious resource. Do you know how you are spending your time? Are you spending your time in a way consistent with furthering your career goals? If not, how much do you really care? What should you be spending more time on? What should you be spending less time on? Do you reflect enough about what you are doing, what you want to accomplish, what you would like to be doing, what you have to learn, how you can beef up that resume?

On Managing Your Career: A Checklist

Yes	No	
_____	_____	Do you know what job you want next, why you want this job?
_____	_____	Have you validated your own assessment of your strengths and weaknesses as a manager?
_____	_____	Do you have or can you obtain a high "emotional intelligence?"
_____	_____	Do you have a plan to significantly improve your resume over the next 12 months?
_____	_____	Do you have a record of "serving" others in your network who can be helpful to your managerial career?
_____	_____	Have you carefully thought about how the rest of your life constrains your career at work, and the extent to which such constraints are truly "givens"?
_____	_____	Are you acting in ways to do more in your present job to help you get your next job?

Practical Exercise

Write a paper on your career objectives and how you plan to achieve them. Begin with an assessment of your current strengths and weaknesses, skills and experience. Next, for a variety of desired jobs, specify the skills and experience required to obtain and excel at the desired positions. Finally, develop a plan to get from where you are to where you want to be, indicating measurable behaviors and temporal milestones. As a second exercise, review your emotional intelligence level, à la Goleman, and validate this with two or three friends. Score yourself as below adequate, adequate, high, or very high. Develop a plan to raise your scores in areas that you are weak, or a plan to adapt your behavior so that you can minimize the adverse consequences of scoring low. For example, you may seek a position where technical skills rather than empathy or social skills are most important.

Afterword

Duncan Neuhauser

Tony Kovner has been my longest-standing coworking professional colleague. We first met in May 1970, at a research conference in Ann Arbor, convened by Basil Georgopolous. This small group included E. Gartly Jaco, Ron Andersen, Edmond Pellegrino, W. Richard Scott, Mayer Zald, Luther Christman, Hans Mauksch, John Griffith, and Fred Munson. The papers presented were published in a book, *Organization Research on Health Institutions* (Georgopolous, 1972), which won the 1974 James A. Hamilton Book Award of the American College of Healthcare Executives. If these names are unfamiliar to you, this is an example of the fleeting nature of academic fame. Professors are known by their publications for a few years, then through their peculiarities and quirks, for the life of their former students, and finally they will be known to an occasional obscure, dust covered historian. By this time only the formal record remains and individual personality is left out of the record. Not here. This book will allow Tony to be remembered as the vivid personality and teacher he is. No one else in the field of health care management in this country has undertaken such an open, personal, honest book-length description of his or her working life. Tony will, by default, stand as representative for this field of health management for this last half century.

I started keeping a personal log book in the Fall of 1970. Here are two quotations from it; first from December 7, 1970:

> *Program Notes AUPHA* came including my appointment to a committee on hospital organization and administration chaired by Professor Charles Frenzel of Duke—this is the first I heard about it.

The first meeting of this task force was held March 15, 1991, at the Association of University Programs in Health Administrative headquarters, One Dupont Circle, Washington, DC.

Tony Kovner . . . was there. He is hard driving, forceful, and intelligent and he tended to push the meeting along so that we got a lot accomplished in terms of going through our agenda.

This task force met for several years and included David Starkweather, Donald Cordes, Paul Gordon, David Luecke, Fred Munson, George Wren, John Champion, and Gary Filerman. This task force reviewed the literature on hospital management used in health management courses across the country and produced a couple of reports (*Association of University Programs*, 1974; Neuhauser, 1972). It appeared there was a need to collect and reprint frequently used articles in one place: a book of readings.

The result was Kovner and Neuhauser's *Health Systems Management: A Book of Readings*, first edition, 1978, and seventh edition due in 2000. This led to a companion *Book of Cases*, first edition, 1981, and sixth edition due in 2000. Rob Fromberg of Health Administration Press estimates that the cumulative sales of both these books through 1998 was 27,000 copies. Only two other health management textbooks have gone through more editions and both of these are now out of print (Berman & various authors).

I see Tony face-to-face on average about two times in three years. Otherwise we talk briefly on the telephone. Here is a typical conversation.

AK: Rob Fromberg thinks it's time for a new edition of our books.
DN: Okay, when?
AK: He wants the manuscript in about six months.
DN: You took the even sections last time. I'll take them this year.
AK: Okay, I'll send you copies of my favorite new articles.
DN: Same here, but you always find more articles than I do. I do have a new teaching case.
AK: Send it to me. So what's new?
DN: (Brief description of a current work-related project)
AK: What a man!
DN: And you?
AK: (Brief description of a current work project) and I have a book for you to read.
DN: (Writes down author and name of book even though I am five years behind in his suggestions) Say hello to Chris for me.
AK: Say hello to Ellie for me. See you.
DN: See you.

That's it. We exchange drafts and comments by mail, the work is done and the next editions are published.

Think of running a successful organization like this for 25 years. For me this is the highest order of organizational efficiency. Hierarchy is oppressive and collegial meetings can take a lot of time. Real efficiency can be achieved when people work toward the same goals with mutual understanding so clear that work-related communication can be minimal, but essential, and the balance of communication can be social and friendly.

This autobiography is both news for me and no surprise, because there are lots of things Tony and I don't talk about. Short of seeing Tony play tennis or his joyous piano playing, the person I have known and worked with for 30 years is to be found in these pages.

While I was writing the history of the American College of Health-care Executives, I became interested in finding biographies or autobiographies of hospital and health care managers in this country in this century (Neuhauser, 1995). I found five and Kovner's is the sixth. Essays written by Henry Hurd, Michael Davis, and Ray Brown are collected in fond memory by friends and colleagues (Blanks, Corely, & Smith, 1972, 1991; Cullen, 1920). George Bugbee wrote the only full-length autobiography. True to his personality, his book is the discreet, unruffled, calm and smooth story of "a good life." This leaves only Ernest Amory Codman's introductory autobiographical chapter in his privately printed book, *The Shoulder* (1934), which is in any way comparable to the book now in your hands.

Without these personal stories, future historians will see health care management as lifeless, wooden, unemotional, and bureaucratic. The passion is removed from the minutes of board meetings and those cryptic business letters that are now being replaced by ephemeral e-mail. But health care managers are real human beings, with feelings of sympathy, and pleasure, who love and hate, get upset, are clever, and make dumb mistakes. We want to make the world a better place, we want to help our families and the next generation of our profession. Thank you, Tony, on behalf of all of us, for telling us your honest story, being a teacher of passion, and caring enough to write this book.

Remembering: Questions

Yes   No

_____   _____   Preserving the historical record of health manage-
                        ment is not my concern

_____ _____ I am content to be known 25 years after my death
                 just as a last name on a large tombstone
_____ _____ I will start a diary

Practical Exercise

Consider a health care organization that you are leading. It is now a hierarchy with supervisors defining and evaluating the work of subordinates. How would you take this hierarchy to a collegial structure where work groups, teamwork, and quality circles are the basis for discussion among equals and become the basis for coordination? Then take this organization to one where only minimal discussion is needed because everyone knows the agreed-upon goal and knows what is needed to get there. How would you do this? (If you need specific examples of such organizations, for the first, think of the military, for the second, a group practice, and the third, a religious denomination without an episcopal hierarchy.)

References

Association of University Programs in Health Administration. (1974, March). *Report of the Task Force on Organization and Administration.* Washington, DC: Author.

Berman, H. J. (1976). *The financial management of hospitals* (3rd ed.). Chicago: Health Administration Press.

Blanks, M. M., Corely, W. E., & Smith, D. S. (Eds.). (1972). *Michael M. Davis: A tribute.* Chicago: Center for Health Administrative Studies, University of Chicago.

Blanks, M. M., Corely, W. E., & Smith, D. S. (Eds.). (1991). *Ray E. Brown: Lectures, messages and memories.* Chicago: Health Administration Press.

Bugbee, G. (1987). *Reflections of a good life: An autobiography.* Chicago: Hospital Research and Education Trust, American Hospital Association.

Burns, J. M. (1978). *Leadership.* New York: Harper Torchbooks.

Chait, R. P., Holland, T. P., & Taylor, B.E. (1991). *The effective board of trustees.* Toronto: Maxwell MacMilllan.

Chait, R. P., Holland, T. P., & Taylor, B. T. (1996). *Improving the performance of the governing board.* Phoenix, AZ: Oryx Press.

Codman, E. A. (1934). *The shoulder.* Boston: Self-printed.

Codman, E. A. (1996). *A study in hospital efficiency.* Oakbrook, IL: Joint Commission on Accreditation of Healthcare Organizations.

Cullen, T. S. (1920). *Henry Mills Hurd: The first superintendent of Johns Hopkins Hospital.* Baltimore, MD: Johns Hopkins University Press.

Cyert, R. M., & March, J. G. (1964). *A behavioral theory of the firm* (pp. 26–43). Englewood Cliffs, NJ: Prentice Hall.

Donabedian, A., et al. (1988). *Medical care chartbook* (7th ed.). Chicago: Health Administration Press.

Drucker, P. F. (1989, July-August). What business can learn from nonprofits. *Harvard Business Review,* pp. 89–93.

Drucker, P. (1999, March–April). Managing oneself. *Harvard Business Review,* pp. 64–75.

Eilers, R. D. (1971). National health insurance: What kind and how much? *New England Journal of Medicine, 284,* 881–886, 945–954.

Freidson, E. (1972). *Profession of medicine.* New York: Dodd Mead.

Georgopolous, B. (Ed.). (1972). *Organization research on health institutions.* Ann Arbor, MI: Institute for Social Research, University of Michigan.

Goleman, D. (1998, Nov.–Dec.). What makes a leader? *Harvard Business Review,* pp. 93–102.

Gordon, P. S. (1961). Top management triangle in voluntary hospitals. *Journal of the Academy of Management, 4,* 205–214.

Gordon, P. S. (1962), Top management triangle in voluntary hospitals. *Journal of the Academy of Management, 5,* 66–75.

Handy, C. (1998). *The hungry spirit.* New York: Broadway Books.

Holland, T. P., Ritvo, R., & Kovner, A. R. (1997). *Improving board effectiveness: Practical lessons for nonprofit health care institutions.* Chicago: American Hospital Publishing.

Jacobs, B. (1981). Role models: Innovations in health care. *New York Affairs, 7,* 79–97.

Jelinek, R., Munson, F., & Smith, R. L. (Eds.). (1977). *SUM: An organizational approach to improved patient care.* Battle Creek, MI: W. K. Kellogg Foundation.

Kindig, D. A., & Kovner, A. R. (Eds.). (1992). *The role of the physician executive: Cases and commentary.* Ann Arbor, MI: Health Administration Press.

Kovner, A. R. (1980). The associate director and the controllers. In A. R. Kovner & D. Neuhauser (Eds.), *Health services management: A book of cases* (2nd ed., pp. 127–139). Chicago: Health Administration Press.

Kovner, A. R. (1986). Reflections on health management education. *Journal of Health Administration Education, 4,* 359–371.

Kovner, A. R. (1988). *Really managing: The work of effective CEOs in large health organizations.* Ann Arbor, MI: Health Administration Press.

Kovner, A. R. (1994a). Community care networks and health care reform: An interview with Robert Sigmund. *Journal of Health Care Administration Education, 12,* 353–372.

Kovner, A. R. (Guest Ed.). (1994b). Community benefit programs for health care organizations. *Journal of Health Administration Education, 12,* 253–288.

Kovner, A. R. (1997). Whose hospital? In A. R. Kovner & D. N. Neuhauser (Eds.), *Health services management* (5th ed.). Chicago: Health Administration Press.

Kovner, A. R., Eilers, R. D., & Kissick, W. (1970, June). *The Penn program in health care administration.* Program notes. Washington, DC: AUPHA.

Kovner, A. R., Kahane, S. B., Katz, G., & Sheps, C. G. (1969, March/April). Relating a neighborhood health center to a hospital: A case history. *Medical Care,* pp. 118–123.

Kovner, A. R., & Neuhauser, D. (Eds.). (1978). *Health services management: Readings and commentary.* Chicago: Health Administration Press.

Kovner, A. R., & Neuhauser, D. (Eds.). (1981). *Health service management: A book of cases.* Chicago: Health Administration Press.

Kovner, A. R., & Neuhauser, D. (Eds.). (1997a). *Health services management:*

Readings and commentary (6th ed.). Chicago: Health Administration Press.

Kovner, A. R., & Neuhauser, D. (Eds.). (1997b). *Health service management: A book of cases* (6th ed.). Chicago: Health Administration Press.

Light, H., & Brown, H. (1967, October). The Gouverneur Health Services Program: An historical view. *Milbank Memorial Fund Quarterly*, pp. 375–389.

Lopez, B. (1986). *Arctic dreams*. New York: Scribner's.

March, J. G., & Simon, H. A. (1958). *Organizations*. New York: John Wiley.

Mechanic, D. (1962). Sources of power of lower participants in complex organizations. *Administrative Sciences Quarterly, 7*, 349–364.

Mintzberg, H. (1983). *Power in and around organizations*. Englewood Cliffs, NJ: Prentice Hall.

Netzer, D. (1981). *The state of the school*. New York: New York University Press.

Neuhauser, D. (1972). *Organizational behavior literature in health administration education*. Washington, DC: Association of University Programs in Health Administration.

Neuhauser, D. (1995). *Coming of age* (60th anniversary ed.). Chicago: Health Administration Press.

Perrow, C. (1963). Goals and power structures: A historical case study. In E. Friedson (Ed.), *The hospital in modern society* (pp. 112–146). New York: Free Press of Glencoe.

Perrow, C. (1984). *Normal accidents: Living with high-risk technology*. New York: Basic Books.

Perrow, C. (1986). *Complex organizations* (3rd ed.). New York: Random House.

Peters, T. (1987). *Thriving in chaos*. New York: Knopf.

Peters, T. (1997). *The circle of innovation*. New York: Knopf.

Pointer, D. D., & Orlikoff, J. E. (1999). *Board work*. San Francisco: Jossey Bass.

Sensenbrenner, J. (1991, March–April). Quality comes to city hall. *Harvard Business Review*, pp. 4–10.

Sofaer, S., et al. (1994). What do we really know about the impact of boards on nonprofit hospital performance? *Journal of Health Administration Education, 9*, 425–442.

Starkweather, D. B. (1970). The rationale for decentralization in larger hospitals. *Hospital Administration, 15*, 27–45.

Strauss, R. (1972). Hospital organization from the viewpoint of patient-centered goals. In B. S. Georgopoulos (Ed.), *Organization research on health institutions* (pp. 203–222). Ann Arbor, MI: Institute for Social Research.

Index

Ackoff, Russell, 131
Adams, George, 99, 139
Advanced Management Program for
    Clinicians (AMPC), 84–87
American College of Health Care
    Executives, 88, 97, 145
American Hospital Association,
    88–90, 106
Anderson, Ron, 145
*The Associate Director and the
    Controllers* (Kovner), 33
Association of University Programs
    of Health Administration,
    97–145
Augustana Nursing Home, 97

Berne, Robert, 127
Blendon, Robert, 79, 82–83
Boufford, Jo Ivey, 60, 127
Brecher, Charles, 117
Brezenoff, Stanley, 108
Brown, Howard, 24, 26, 28
Brown, Ray, 147
Bugbee, George, 147
Burns, James M., 5

Career management, 137–138
Chait, Richard, 105–108
Champion, John, 146
Christman, Luther, 145
Codman, Ernest, 147
Commonwealth Foundation (The), 79
Complex Organizations (Perrow), 23
Community benefit programs, 91

Connors, Edward, 88
Cordes, Donald, 145
Cornell University, Graduate School
    of Business and Public
    Administration, 19–20
Cyert, Richard, 48

Davis, Michael, 147
Delgado, Jane, 88
DeTorynay, Rheba, 81
DeVries, Robert, 84, 86
Diversity, 35–38
Doctoral education, 123
Drucker, Peter, 51, 98

Education
    for health care management,
        44–46, 119–126
    on teaching, 47–49, 51–54
The Effective Board of Trustees
    (Chait, Holland,
    & Taylor), 106
Eilers, Robert, 39–45, 60, 124
Etzioni, Amitai, 106

Filerman, Gary, 146
Finkler, Steven, 118, 124
First Professional Bank, 97
Filerman, Gary, 146
For-profits, 1, 20–22
Foundations, 77–96
Freidson, Eliot, 92
Frenzel, Charles, 145
Fromberg, Rob, 146

Glasser, Melvin, 56, 59–61
Gordon, Paul, 146
Gouverneur Health Services Program
    (GHSP), 23–38, 48
Governance
    Anytown Hospital, 70–73
    board retreats, 108
    College of Physicians, 102–103
    Health System, 103–105
    information for the board, 93
    lack of accountability, 92
    lessons learned, 2–6
    Lutheran Medical Center, 108–110
    Management and Organizational
        Evaluation Committee,
        109–110
    Nominations and Board
        Development Committee,
        209
    nonprofit, 97–113
    readiness, 112
    study of New Jersey Hospitals,
        49–51
    University, 101–102
Graduate School of Public
    Administration (see Wagner
    School and NYU)
Grant, Christine, 79
Griffith, John, 145

Handy, Charles, 75, 141
Hattis, Paul, 88, 90
Health Services Management:
    A Book of Readings (Kovner
    & Neuhauser), 146
Health Services Management:
    A Book of Cases (Kovner
    & Neuhauser), 146
Hemingway, Ernest, 93
Hofmann, Paul, 88
Holland, Thomas, 97, 103, 106–108
Hospital Community Benefit
    Standards Program, 87–92
Hunts Point Home, 14–18

Hurd, Henry, 147

Improving Board Effectiveness (Holland,
    Ritvo, & Kovner), 106
Improving the Performance of the
    Governing Board (Chait,
    Holland, & Taylor), 106

Jaco, E. Gartly, 145
Jacobs, Barry, 98
Job search, 76–77
Joint Commission on Accreditation
    of Health Care Organizations
    (JCAHO), 87, 90, 100

Kellogg Foundation (The WKK), 79,
    84–87, 99
Kindig, David, 85
Kissick, William, 44–45
Knickman, James, 118, 124
Kovner, Anthony, R.
    in academia, 115–135
    eight careers, 6–8
    family business, 11–22
    family history, 8–9
    governance study, 49–51
    hospital chief executive, 67–77
Kovner, Harold, 11–12
Kovner, Sidney, 11–12, 16–18
Kovner, Victor, 11–12
Kropf, Roger, 118, 121

Learning (and lessons)
    about myself, 17–18
    health care delivery for the poor,
        31–32
    from HCBSP, 90–92
    from my father, 16–17
    from your parents, 9–10
    at Penn, 46–50
    at the UAW, 62–65
    about teaching, 123–124
Light, Harold, 24, 26, 28
Lilly Endowment, 97, 103, 105

Luecke, David, 146
Lutheran Medical Center, 97–100,
    139
  governance, 108–110

Maimonides Medical Center, 108
Management
  in academia, 39–54, 115–132
  appraising performance, 75–77
  between life and work, 138–139
  effective health care manager,
    139–140
  of a faculty, 128–138
  as hospital chief executive, 67–77
  lessons learned, 1–2
  as program director, 118–119
  services for the poor, 23–38
  teaching, 124–126
  working with physician managers,
    131–133
  your career, 137–138
March, James, 19, 48
Martin, Samuel, 80
Mauksch, Hans, 145
McClelland, Richard, 106
Mechanic, David, 48
Metropolitan Health Plan, 97
Mintzberg, Henry, 98
Mount Sinai Hospital, 11, 115
Mount Sinai NYU Health System,
    128–130
Munson, Fred, 145–146

National health insurance, 6–7,
    42–44, 61–62, 73, 93
Netzer, Dick, 115–119
Neuhauser, Duncan, 125, 145
Newman, Howard, 41
New York Affairs, 98–99
New York University (NYU), 6, 85,
    89, 94, 115–116, 120
  Stern School of Business,
    129–130
Nonprofits, (*see* Governance)

Normal Accidents (Perrow), 23

Organizations (March & Simon), 19
*Organization Research on Health
    Institutions* (Georgopoulos),
    145
Orlikoff, James, 2

Padilla, Elena, 117
Park East Hospital, 11–12
Pelligrino, Edmond, 145
Pennsylvania (University of)
  managing in academia, 39–54
  Wharton School, 117
Perrow, Charles, 23, 48
Peters, Tom, 76
Pew Charitable Trusts, 79
Physician managers, 131–135
Pittsburgh (University of), 23
Pointer, Dennis, 2

Reflections on Management Education
    (Kovner), 119
Relman, Arnold, 39–40
Richardson, Hila, 81
Ritvo, Roger, 97, 103
Robert Wood Johnson Foundation
    (The), 79–84, 118, 140
Rodwin, Victor, 83, 86, 118
Rogers, David, 80, 82–83
Rosenberg, Marv, 30, 33
Rural hospitals
  program of extended care, 79–82
  hospital-based program, 82–84

Schall, Ellen, 121
Scott, W. Richard, 145
Sensenbrenner, J., 64
Sheps, Cecil G., 23–24, 31–32, 34
The Shoulder (Codman), 147
Sigmond, Robert, 87–91
Simon, Herbert, 19
Smith, Howard, 99, 108
Sofaer, Shoshona, 98

Sparks, John, 60
Starkweather, David, 48, 146
Strauss, Robert, 48
Swing beds, 81–82

Taylor, Barbara, 106–108
Teaching, 123–126
Thier, Samuel, 39, 80, 88
Trussell, Ray, 34

Union, 51–65
United Autoworkers Union (UAW),
    51–65

Vladeck, Bruce, 88

Wagner School (Robert F. Wagner
    Graduate School of Public
    Service at NYU), 99,
    115–135
Weitzman, Beth, 118
White, Rodney, 19, 23
Wren, George, 146

Yedidia, Michael, 118

Zald, Mayer, 145